IF IT HURTS
DON'T STRETCH IT

A Guide to Understanding How Common Aches and Pains Occur and the Frequent Misconceptions Around How to Treat Them

Adam Dowsett

Grosvenor House
Publishing Limited

This book is published by
Grosvenor House Publishing Ltd
Link House
140 The Broadway, Tolworth, Surrey, KT6 7HT.
www.grosvenorhousepublishing.co.uk

A CIP record for this book
is available from the British Library

ISBN 978-1-83975-861-4
eBook ISBN 978-1-80381-091-1

Dedication

This book is dedicated to my amazing and supportive
wife Sara and to my new baby boy Jack.
I love you guys.

Contents

Preface

The human body is fascinating. It's incredible to think about all the physical processes that are happening day in and day out just to keep us functioning. Most of these we take for granted and most happen without any conscious thought on our part. Everything is great until there's a glitch in the system and we experience pain. Pain is the brain's way of telling us that something is under stress but rarely does it tell us why. There are obvious examples where it's not too tricky to work out what's going on. If you bump your shin on the end of the bed it hurts. There has been a clear trauma to a specific point and pain duly follows. But I've always been more interested in the pains that don't seem to have an obvious source. Why does your neck just ache sometimes? You can't remember knocking it, overworking it, overtraining it or stressing it. You haven't done anything different so why would it hurt? What do you do with this pain? How do you make it go away? Stretching it feels nice temporarily but it doesn't really make the pain go away long-term. You get a little window of improvement, maybe seconds, minutes or hours but then the pain comes back. Why? This is what I found fascinating as a child and still do to this day. Let me describe my experiences that lead me to choose my career and then to write this book.

I first started getting significant neck and back pain from around the age of ten. At primary school it would be sore and uncomfortable just to sit on the floor in assembly. At secondary school I'd be in considerable pain by 9am after simply being stood in assembly for half an hour and then that would stay with me throughout the day in each lesson at school. It always seemed to ease off if I ran around at lunchtime but would always hurt again as soon as I sat back down again for the afternoon. When the pain was at its worst and I didn't know how to get comfortable or make it better, I would just lie on the couch or in bed after getting home from school. My neck would regularly go into spasm for no apparent reason. I was about twelve years old when my neck completely locked up after the extreme action of heading a balloon. Now, through my knowledge and experience, I can look back and understand why these things happened to me but at the time it was scary as you start to wonder, "If I'm getting these issues now what am I going to be like when I'm older?" Because of the uncomfortable feelings in my back and neck I'd be quite fidgety and would struggle to sit or stand straight as I couldn't hold myself in basic postural positions. Now, writing this at the age of 34, I can work a full day on my feet all day long and have absolutely zero back pain every day. But to get here I had to go through a process, which initially regularly included doing the wrong things, to work out how to manage my own body.

Prior to the balloon incident I'd already started having treatment to try and help my neck and back. I saw a variety of people, with varying degrees of success but there was always a common theme. I was always told to stretch my neck and stretch my back. Without fail my 'homework' always included some form of neck stretch and lower back stretch. Initially, I followed all the advice as I wanted to be a good kid and do my homework but after a couple of years of not getting anywhere I started to question things. I was stuck in a cycle and was just going around in circles. The odd day here and there of being pain-free didn't seem to justify all the work of doing the stretches. So, I decided I'd do little experiments where I'd have periods of not doing the stretches and to my surprise I'd get little improvements. We're talking minor improvements but it got me thinking *why when I don't stretch the bit that hurts do I feel a bit better?* This then led to the question, *is there something I should be stretching instead?* By this point I was around fourteen. I'd lit a spark of interest and been able to get my pain levels tolerable enough that I could manage day-to-day activities. At that point, I'd just played the first injury free full football season since I could remember so I was a happy lad!

For the next few years, up until the age of twenty, I remained curious about how the body worked but, as I was managing to stay relatively pain-free in comparison to previous years, I hadn't explored my curiosities any further. That was until I started getting some pain in my left knee in preseason football training. The pain started as slight discomfort below the knee in July but progressively worsened until by January of the following year I couldn't run, jump or kick without feeling significant discomfort. Looking back of course I should have gone to get some advice much sooner but I thought it would sort itself out if I tried resting it or that if I ignored it enough it would just go away. In my head I hadn't done anything to my knee that I could pinpoint the pain to at all. Remembering my previous issues with my back and neck I tentatively tried stretching it and, although I immediately felt relief, I quickly realised it actually made the problem worse. A soft tissue therapist had been recommended to me so I faced the situation and visited her knowing full well that when I said football made it worse she'd recommend I stop playing. I knew she was right but I didn't want to hear it. I was fascinated by her approach to connecting the dots. After a few tests, a lot of digging into my history and some treatment we'd got to the issue. The long and short of it was that I had patella tendonitis, caused by five separate quadricep tears I'd had over the past four years, which I'd forgotten about. These were caused by the tight left hip flexor muscles, which were tight because I had always leant on my right leg, due to a weak right glute. My back pain had always been on my right side but I'd always been given lower back stretching for both sides. If the right side of my lower back was already overstretched from leaning on that leg, had I been making it worse by stretching it more? As part of my work now I refer to 'connecting the dots' or the 'flow diagram' of working out the process of why your symptom started every day.

My initial spark of interest had now become a flame. My wife Sara (who was my girlfriend at the time) could see how intrigued I was and encouraged me to do the same course as the therapist I'd seen. The therapist herself also encouraged me but I didn't quite have the courage at the time to make the leap. This is where the universe stepped in. After six months of rehabilitation, along with a bit of preseason training, I was ready to play football again. The tendon felt 100% and I felt pretty good fitness wise. I was ready and the time had come. I ran on as a second-half substitute and within 10 minutes I'd scored. I should've been delighted, celebrating the result of all my hard work and effort through the rehabilitation process. In reality I was lying in a crumpled heap on the floor with a broken tibia and fibula where I'd collided with the goalkeeper in the process of scoring. That wasn't part of the plan.

After an operation, a few days in hospital, time off from my job due to the injury and a realisation of how much work I was going to need to do for this rehabilitation, I decided this must have been a sign that I should start my soft tissue therapist training. I signed up for the next available course and started my training the following year. It remains one of the best decisions I've ever made. The trainers were fantastic and through understanding the dot-to-dot process further, I was able to piece together how and why I'd had the issues I'd had as a youngster. Understanding what had happened when I was younger couldn't change my past but it confirmed that there was a lot of hope for the future. I felt and still feel now that being able to understand how things function and where they can go wrong is priceless. However, as my clients will testify, I am regularly heard saying that looking after yourself is an ongoing process. This may sound negative and not what you want to hear but you're never really completely 'fixed'. You'll never make it to a place where you don't need to look after yourself. It may be a harsh reality but it's true. I find the easiest comparison here is nutrition. You wouldn't expect to be able to eat whatever you want, whenever you want and everything feel great. There would understandably be consequences due to the amount and quality of fuel that you put into your system. The musculoskeletal system is no different in that it responds to how you use it. The tricky part, which again parallels nutrition, is that the reactions aren't often instant. If you eat a takeaway you don't feel immediately full or groggy. If you look down at your new phone/tablet while curled up on the sofa your neck doesn't hurt the second you look down. But in both of these scenarios, along with thousands of others, it's the compounding snowball effect of repeated stresses to the system that eventually lead to a response. Using the neck scenario the response may well be waking up one morning, maybe a few weeks later, with a very stiff or sore neck thinking, "I must have slept funny because I don't remember doing anything." The aim of this book is to get you to think about how you use your body every day and not just pay attention to it when something has gone wrong (which we can all be guilty of). Also, when you have discomfort in your body in the future, being able to understand why it is happening can lead you to stretching the actual area that needs the attention, which is often not the area causing the discomfort and asking for attention. For example, if you've spent all day gardening, leaning forward and reaching out in front of you, when your lower back hurts as you get up why do you really want to lean forward, try and touch your toes and stretch your back out even more? When you do stretch forward why, at that point, does it feel nice to do so, even though it's actually adding more stress to the area?

Step-by-step this book will cover the most common issues that we all face and that I see in my practice most frequently. Unfortunately, I have to stress this point, as I will throughout this book, that this is not a 'one-size-fits-all' approach. There is no 'normal' or 'average' person but I have found the concepts that we will cover do relate to the vast majority of people. Also, this isn't designed to get everyone to self-diagnose themselves so please seek professional advice if you're unsure on anything. Hopefully, it will prove to be a useful reference for you and get you to think differently about pain, why we have it and what we can do about it.

Before we move on I want to go back to the point about never being 'fixed'. When I say this to clients it often gets a negative response, understandably I think. Sometimes I'm met with, "I thought I was paying you to fix me." The point is that we have to work on keeping ourselves in a balanced place. Be it physically, psychologically or nutritionally, there are numerous areas in the body that need regular attention to keep the entire system working. And here comes another downer – we're not indestructible. You can do all the right things and yet things can still go wrong.

I had another 'useful' experience five years ago that I want to tell you about. It was four months before we were due to get married, I was feeling fit and strong and had just got into playing badminton with a few friends. We'd play once a week and, although we'd only been playing for four or five weeks, I was really getting into it. Sara was happy as I'd stopped playing football a few months before because I didn't want to risk getting injured before the wedding. I picked badminton as it's a non-contact sport and a really good form of exercise. You can probably see where this is going by now. Our hour was nearly up on the court and we'd played a few sets of some cracking badminton doubles. I'm not sure if this is entirely true but I'll say it was the deciding set to add to the drama. I jumped up for a smash and missed it – gutting. But more gutting was the fact that as I landed, with no contact from anyone else, no slip or twist, my right ankle dislocated and broke. My shin was at 12o'clock but my foot was at 2o'clock. To this day I don't have a reason for what happened but that's why I refer to it as a 'useful' experience. I know I was possibly the strongest and most aligned I'd ever been. When I was younger I used to go over on my ankles frequently but I hadn't had any issues for years. Ironically, the day before, I was talking to a client about how good my ankles were now because I was aligned and that she needn't worry because we'd get her to that place soon as well. But as I know my alignment and functionality were really good at that time, I just have to put it down to being human. We're not exact, precise machines. That's why I have to emphasise that the ideas in this book can't stop you ever getting injured again. Nothing and no one can. However, if you can get everything functioning in and around the areas to the best of their abilities, you can greatly reduce the risks. Another upside is the fact that, if you do get unlucky, with a good functional base then you will recover quicker. For me, although my ankle injury was a lot worse than the broken leg a few years before, I recovered much quicker as my body, mind and level of knowledge at the time of injury were in a better place.

Acknowledgements

Starting at the beginning I need to thank my first soft tissue therapist, Claire Day, for helping me not just to understand my own body better and helping fix my issues but also for inspiring me to pursue a career in this area.

That encouragement led me to studying at the London School of Sports Massage. I'd like to thank all my tutors there for teaching and inspiring me to start and continue to learn and develop my skills as a therapist.

I couldn't have developed those skills without clients. I'm grateful to every client that I have seen over the years and for every client that I will see in the future for giving me the opportunity to practise and develop my skills, while always learning something new from every single one of you.

These experiences led me to write this book but you wouldn't be reading it now if it wasn't for the help of everyone at Grosvenor House Publishing who took it from being an idea to reality. I'm not blessed artistically so I also need to thank Keirone Capstack for all his work in creating the illustrations for this book.

Finally, I want to acknowledge the impact on my life of a late friend, Steve Bernard. Steve was a great friend who tragically passed away at the age of just 18 years. I'm grateful for how he inspired me as a friend both before and after his passing and he remains a strong motivator in much of what I do in my life. His legacy continues through the Steve Bernard Foundation (you can find out more at www.stevebernardfoundation.com) and by purchasing this book you are helping the foundation with a percentage of profits going towards the charity as they continue to do amazing work.

Introduction

Firstly, thank you for buying this book. I really hope you find it a useful guide for helping you to look after yourself. I hope it gets you thinking about how your body is constantly working in everything you do and how subtle changes here and there can make a massive difference to your life.

I work as a soft tissue therapist and have been doing so for over 10 years now. Over the years I have predominantly worked seeing clients in my own clinic but have also worked at two other clinics, as well as a premier league football club. It's always fascinated me how interconnected the body is and how a slight glitch at one point in the network can have such a major impact elsewhere. Over the years of treating hundreds of clients of all ages and athletic abilities, who undertake a massive range of jobs, hobbies and activities, I've learned that one thing is for sure — we are all complex beings and there isn't a 'one-size-fits-all' approach to dealing with the human body.

However, this book will cover the most common issues that we face in modern life and what I believe are the best ways that you can approach and overcome these challenges. I've seen it work for hundreds of clients so far, of all ages and abilities and I am passionate about getting these messages to as many people as possible. I'm also a realist. When I was a kid I fell from a climbing frame and landed on my wrist. Gravity and concrete won on that occasion and I broke my arm. Good posture and loose hamstrings weren't going to save me on that day. So many common aches and pains, both acute and chronic, can have relatively simple causes and, accordingly, fixes that are often less complicated than expected. That's what excites me about this job. Every client I see and speak to is an individual project. There's no other you in the world. No one else has lived your life, had your experiences, your thoughts or your actions and that's why there can't be a generic approach to your body. However, there are many things that we all tend to have in common. The majority of us tend to look down more than we look up throughout the day, so what does that mean for the muscles of the neck? We tend to do more with our arms in front of us rather than behind us so how does that affect the muscles of the shoulders and upper back? This book aims to get you thinking about how your body functions in your everyday activities and not just when you're exerting yourself in exercise or sport, although we will be covering lots of those activities as well.

The preface covered a bit of my personal history that led me to become interested in this area and also eventually led me to work in the field and discover the concepts and patterns that have helped hundreds of clients so far and which will hopefully help you too. Although it essentially showed a selection from my injury autobiography, this book isn't just me wanting to tell you about my injuries. I hope that having an idea of what I've been through, seen and done will hopefully resonate with you. I'm coming at this from a real-life experience perspective rather than a 'textbook scenario' because, like I've already suggested, there isn't a 'normal' or 'average' person. We are all unique and fascinating and have our own stories. I've been in that place where I genuinely wondered whether I was going to be stuck with the pain forever and had thoughts such as, "I'm doing what I'm supposed to be doing so why isn't it getting better?" As I'm sure many of you will have experienced, that's not a nice place to be. I've got to be honest with you here – I'm not going to claim that anything is a magic fix, or that if you do a certain exercise once a day forever you'll be cured because that just isn't true. Having and maintaining a healthy, functional body is an ongoing process involving ups and downs. When it's going great you feel invincible. When you're in pain it sucks. I firmly believe that with a bit of knowledge and a good toolbox of ideas you'll find that, more often than not, you can relieve your pain and, maybe more importantly, keep yourself out of pain and in the best place you can be.

The concepts covered in this book include the most common issues that I see in my practice. It would be an epic tale if I attempted to cover every niggle or injury I've come across at work and the cocktail of causes that have led to each and every one of those. But I'm pretty confident you will have experienced at least a few of these over your lifetime, so hopefully this book will help you to understand a bit more about why it could have happened, what to do about it if it happened again and, more importantly, how best to avoid it happening again. Too many of us have been told that we've got an issue that we'll have just have to learn to live with, that we'll have learn to manage the pain or that all that's left is to rely on painkillers to get through the day. Whether that's a chronic issue that nobody can work out the cause of, a recurring issue that you think has finally gone but then comes back to bite you out of nowhere or a new pain that's seemingly appeared unexpectedly, there are a chain of events that have to have occurred for it to happen. If you can have an idea of what that chain might look like then you've got at least a fighting chance of being able to alter and manage that chain. It's a horrible feeling when you feel helpless and almost controlled by pain. Anyone who's had their lower back go into spasm and experienced the horrendous pain and almost scary restriction in movement will know how vulnerable it can make you feel. Pain isn't fun. Be the pain short-term or long-term, it causes stress on the body and it's the body's way of telling you something needs to change. With some things the body is awesome at protecting itself. For example, if you touch something hot your reflexes are amazing at getting your hand away from the danger. Well played body. However, in many cases we experience pain seemingly without a cause. Why did your back go into spasm putting the lead on the dog on Monday morning? It didn't happen when you did it Sunday night. It's never happened the hundreds of times before when you've done it. The body doesn't give you a printout or summary for its reasons – you're just in pain. Why, when you were out for a walk on some nice flat, smooth ground did you go over on your ankle? Where did that come from? It can be quite confusing, as well as annoying, because if you knew it was going to happen then you'd avoid it but what could you have done differently?

Of course, using my broken wrist as a prime example, sometimes we do just get unlucky. If you're out for a run in the winter, slip on some ice and fall on your knee then your knee is going to hurt. That one doesn't need too much investigating on my part but next is an example of something I see more frequently. So, say you're out for a run as normal and towards the end of that run your right knee starts to ache a bit. Then, over the weeks it starts to ache increasingly, not enough to stop you yet but it's definitely talking to you a bit more and you think, "Maybe I'll have a week off. Maybe I'm doing too much." So, you have your week off, the pain seems to have gone, you go back out and the pain's still there. Maybe it's your shoes. They're not that old but it could be worth trying to change them. Begrudgingly, you part with a fair chunk of change to get the new shoes. Have they done the trick? No? Nightmare. This is when I normally get a call saying, "My knee hurts running, I've tried resting and new shoes and it didn't work. It's probably just that I'm running too much. Someone I know sees you. Can you help me?" Obviously, in a perfect world this made-up person would already have had an assessment and treatment beforehand to make sure that their body was ready for running, in terms of functionality and alignment and the whole issue could probably have been avoided. The reality is that, over all the years of seeing clients, I've only ever had **three** people who've come in and said, "Nothing's wrong. I haven't had any injuries before but you see a few people I know and I just want to check I'm ok." These people get gold stars but the reality for nearly all of us, myself included in the past, is that we don't tend to get support until an issue has happened. If we go back to the made-up example, after they've explained a bit of the background I will usually say something like, "If it was just simply a case that you were just running too much then both knees would hurt." That's normally met with silence for a couple of seconds and then, "Oh, I hadn't thought about it like that." If it were purely the impact or distance or stress of running then both knees would be feeling the strain the same, so if only one side is giving you discomfort then that's an immediate clue that something is out of alignment which can hopefully be realigned. I've got so many clients who were told they'd never do a certain activity again due to their 'dodgy' ankle/knee/back that have been able to return to that activity again by maximising the functionality of their bodies. It's awesome that they can get aligned enough, strong enough and confident enough to do that.

Throughout this book I will give numerous examples of the most common issues I see and the best recommended resolutions to these. As I said earlier it would be impossible to cover every known issue and injury but hopefully there are at least one or two with which you can resonate.

CHAPTER 1

Common Challenges

We are all unique. As I said earlier no one else has lived your life, had your experiences, your thoughts or your actions. The stresses and strains that your body has been through are different to any other person on the planet. The stresses and strains you're currently putting your body through may be very different to what you were doing 10 years ago and are likely to be very different to what you'll be doing in another 10 years' time. We're talking about day-to-day activities, posture, sports, exercise – everything you do. As the world develops, the activities/jobs/sports/exercise we do, as well as technology, all develop too. Three hundred years ago the seat position in your car wasn't something you had to think about. One hundred years ago ensuring you had a correct desk setup at work wasn't on many people's radar. Nor was thinking about how much your screen time could be affecting you. Who knows what the future holds for things like this. It maybe in another 50 years' time some of the challenges I refer to as 'common' today won't even exist anymore but however things develop one thing is for sure – you will always have to look after you and you will always be using your body every day for your whole life. Even if in 30 years' time you're doing a job that hasn't even been invented yet you will still be using your body so having that awareness of what you're doing and how you're using your body is a lifelong gift.

There might be some people out there who have been doing the same job for the last 10 years and plan to do it again for the next 10 years in an industry where not many changes occur. So, for them it could be easy to think that as not much has or is going to change for them that maybe they don't need to focus as much. Firstly, complacency is a dangerous thing for our bodies. Having set routines or being on autopilot isn't often a good thing. If something in our routine is the tiniest bit off, that will multiply day-by-day and week-by-week, often in the background without us consciously knowing and this exponential growth can eventually lead to a much bigger issue. This is where the snowball effect is at its strongest as by just ticking over and getting by we think our bodies are ok and that's when we seemingly get an issue unexpectedly. Secondly, although your job may be the same over this 20 year period how about the rest of your life? There's literally hundreds of areas we could look at here so I'm going to pick just a few out. Over that 20 years would you have had the same mattress, sofa or car; done the same sports/activities; had exactly the same levels of stress? If the answer is yes to some of these then these may still be different to how they were 20 years ago. If the answer is no, then things will definitely have changed, meaning you would have had to adapt to the changes. This point isn't designed to make people overanalyse or become obsessive about how they are using their body every second of every day. A case in point for this is sleep. Often clients will tell me that they think they don't sleep in a good position and, if this does seem relevant to their issues, we try and adapt things as best we can. However, you can't truly control how you sleep. For example, if someone has a bad neck and, once we work out what the issue is, it seems that sleeping on their front looking the same way may be contributing, we will always discuss trying to train them into sleeping in a different position. But, if they sleep on their front because sleeping any other way would cause terrible back pain that wakes them up in the night then you have a decision to make about what to prioritise. In reality, as everything in the body is interlinked, we would inevitably look at trying to sort both issues through treatment, stretches and exercises. But let's say it's just a neck issue for now, is it realistic to just start sleeping on your back instead with a perfectly neutral head position? You could try going to sleep like that but chances are you wouldn't get to sleep as the body has gotten used to sleeping on the front. Even if you did get off to sleep you'd probably wake up either in the night or in the morning back on your front again.

We're creatures of habit and we don't have a reset button unfortunately. You'd be a very rich person if you could find a way to magically put a person into a perfect posture with perfect strength. But what is perfect anyway? All we can do is our best to try and make our bodies work the best that they can. I remember when I started my training I thought I was going to be dealing with all the acute injuries. I thought it was going to be a revolving door of back spasms, muscle tears, twisted ankles, you name it. The reality is that over the years of seeing clients I would say at least 95% of people who come through the door have an issue that would be classed as chronic. Even those who come in bent in two with their back in spasm will have a history or it won't be the first time that it has spasmed. I do see issues and injuries that are random (I've had a couple myself) and seemingly unexplained and/or unlucky but these are very much the minority. Over the years I've had clients that, among many other things, have slipped on surfaces and twisted their knees, gone over on a rock and twisted their ankle or picked up something heavier than they thought it was and hurt their back. These things do happen and any injury is unfortunate. Most of those situations that I can remember have happened to existing clients who were in a good place before it happened so again, although frustrating for them and for me, the only bright side is that they recover quicker than average because they were pretty strong and balanced in the first place.

However, most clients do come in with issues that have been nagging them for weeks, months, maybe even years. My first experience of soft tissue therapy came around because I decided to do something because the issue didn't go away by itself and I'd been in pain for six months. We can all be guilty of leaving things and hoping they settle down by themselves, so this isn't a criticism. I make a point of never telling a new client they should have come in sooner because that won't change anything. The only time I do get frustrated is if an existing client has the knowledge and doesn't do anything about it (for example, they come once a month for maintenance treatment but they twist their ankle between sessions and don't contact me as they don't want to bother me before the next session) because for some issues getting treatment as soon as possible is important. However, thankfully this is a rarity as I always talk to clients about how everything is interlinked and how a glitch in one part of the network will affect the network as a whole.

Back to the chronic issues and, more often than not, a client won't have a specific thing they can put their finger on that has caused an issue. The reason for this is again, more often than not, because there isn't a single cause and it's usually a combination of numerous factors that culminate to result in a stress in the network. These factors will usually come from all parts of life and, although a certain activity at work or movement in a sport may exacerbate the pain, there's usually a few dots in the dot-to-dot that need addressing.

It wouldn't be realistic to think of every possible movement that could cause stress on your body and write about how we manage these as this would be the longest book ever written. What I've tried to do though is look at specific areas of the body, the biggest challenges we face there and the most common issues I see. You'll see as you read on that although there's a separate neck and upper back section, this will often interlink with shoulders. I'm not trying to get you to think of body parts in isolation by separating them into their sections. It's quite the opposite but I think it's the best way of trying to break things down. I've written this book in such a way that if in a few years' time you had a random pain in your elbow you would hopefully think, "I won't stretch it until I've had a think about what I've been up to." You could maybe flick to the section on the elbow for ideas.

However, I would encourage you to read the whole book because you never know what's round the corner and hopefully by having a greater insight into how things are so interlinked and knowing that pain is just the symptom at the end of the chain, you may be able to make changes in areas you hadn't even thought about before that will save you from future pain. Your future self will love you for it.

I'd love to be able to say I could stop you getting injured. I'd love it if there was a way we could make ourselves indestructible. Having your body working the best it can is the closest I think you can get to that. If this book gets you to think differently about how you use your body then it's worked. Like I said earlier this isn't about you trying to figure everything out for yourself and sometimes, however hard you look at it, some things don't get figured out. But if you can make a few, or even a lot of, minor changes which allow you to have more enjoyment out of your body then that's awesome. If you're not sure why something is hurting and this inspires you to see someone for help after a few days instead of a couple of months because things don't 'sort themselves out' then that's awesome too as you could well have saved yourself weeks or even months of pain and potential future injuries.

CHAPTER 2

The Concept

Hopefully, even if you hadn't thought about it before, by now you're thinking how interconnected everything in the body is and how a minor change in one area can have a much bigger impact elsewhere. With this in mind there simply can't be a blanket approach to every physical pain we have. Painkillers can't be the answer for everything. Neither can exercising your way through the pain or simply ignoring the pain and hoping it goes away. Speaking to someone who claims that there is an answer for everything, isn't the answer either.

I'm going to share with you the four main principles that I work by. I'm not claiming they provide the answer for everything but these principles have helped hundreds of people to get out and for many stay out of pain, so I want to share them in the hope that they will help you too.

Before sharing these principles I want to get you to think about the similarities between physical pain and psychological pain. This will all make sense in a minute but I want you to think about a time when something made you really mad but it was actually not that big of a deal. Was it in the car the other day when someone was outrageously rude by not saying thank you to you when you let them go? Was it someone breathing really loudly next to you on the train? Was it shouting at that person who cut in front of you in the queue? Was it that dog barking when you were trying to get to sleep? You get the idea. At that moment in time you can literally feel the rage bubbling up inside you. You're ready to explode and sometimes we do explode in those times. You might surprise yourself at how angry you felt or how you reacted. You might wonder where that rage came from. For many it may be out of character, for some maybe not but however you look at the act itself (e.g. someone cutting in front of you) in reality it probably didn't need to provoke the reaction it did. Once the dust has settled most of us will realise it wasn't actually really about that person cutting in front of us. We were actually really annoyed about something that had happened earlier that day or maybe even the day or week before. On another day, if everything were ok on the day that someone cut in front of you, you might not have even noticed or you may have just rolled your eyes or told them that you were there first and they would have apologised and gone behind you. We might not work it out immediately but usually in the end we can appreciate that although we did get angry at a situation it was actually more about something else that was going on for us and the anger was just the issue coming out in a different setting. We don't just take it at face value that we now have an anger problem and are going to be angry forever. We can be curious about what's really going on and explore the chain of events that lead us to the place where we snapped at the queue jumper.

Generally, I don't think we do this enough with physical pain. I think it's too easy to say back pain means you have a bad back. Getting angry about something once doesn't mean you have an anger management issue so why should having a pain in your knee mean you've now got a knee issue? This takes us to the first principle.

Pain is just the symptom

I can't emphasise enough how different this is to 'pain is where the problem is'. Pain occurs where the network is most under stress. Very rarely are the cause and the symptom the same. Of course, there are examples such as dropping something heavy on your toe, where the chain of events is short and simple and that's why you have pain. But for the vast majority of scenarios pain is just the symptom at the end of a series of events. Throughout this book we'll cover countless examples of this process in action. This is a very significant principle to start with as hopefully it gets you thinking about pain in a different way. That's why I like to link it to psychology as, over the years, I've seen so many people struggle for weeks, months, years, even decades being told they have the metaphorical equivalent of 'anger management issues'. Countless clients have been told that they're going to be stuck with their bad 'x' forever, yet all the X-rays, MRI's and blood tests have told them that there's nothing wrong with 'x'. So, they're left with feeling pain in an area that they're frequently being told there's nothing wrong with and, to rub salt into the wound, they're told it can't be sorted. These are classic examples of pain just being the symptom. The reason nothing can be found on the tests is because that's not where the issue is – it's just the symptom.

At times it can seem like the brain is playing tricks on you. A classic example of this is when people have neck pain. The brain will tell you that your neck feels stiff or stuck and that you need to free it up. For many that then takes the form of rolling or stretching or clicking the neck in some way so that you get that 'release'. I used to do this when I was a kid as I thought it was helping because at that deepest point of the stretch it would feel so nice. Most of us know a friend or relative that's always clicking or twisting their neck. But would they ever stop to think about why they're always needing to do it? If it did give them the relief that they thought they were getting by clicking or stretching their neck then surely they wouldn't need to do it again. Once again this emphasises that, in most cases, focusing solely on the symptom isn't the answer. In this specific scenario, at best, you get some temporary relief but in reality you're just firefighting the symptom while there is a bigger underlying imbalance at play. This links us nicely to the next principle.

If it hurts don't stretch it

That's right. If it hurts don't stretch it. Many people challenge me on this because, as we alluded to earlier, the brain is often telling you to stretch the bit that hurts. Using the neck example again it can actually feel nice to stretch the neck when you're doing it but does it actually need stretching? As an estimate I'd say that in about 95% of cases it's important not to stretch the area that hurts. As always, there are examples where this isn't the case, most notably when you get cramp. That is the main obvious exception to this principle and on rare occasions there are specific examples where you do need to stretch what hurts but I'll repeat that in about 95% of cases stretching should be avoided in the area where there is pain. Not only that but, in most cases, stretching the area that is sore actually makes things worse. I could list hundreds of examples here but I think it's important to understand why it is so important not to stretch the area that hurts.

The best way to visualise this is to imagine you've got a bit of Blu Tack. It's a new bit so it's solid and strong. This new bit of Blu Tack models your muscle in a strong state at its optimum length. There's no stress on it and if you imagine the nerves running through the muscles then there'd be no stress on them either. If the nerves are stress free then you won't have a need for a stress response and no pain is felt. Easy. However, if you took hold of each end of the Blu Tack and slowly began to pull them away from each other, then the Blu Tack would start to stretch and lengthen. You can also visualise the nerves inside the Blu Tack muscle also beginning to stretch and lengthen. Now we're starting to put the nerves under a bit of stress so they'd now be starting to respond and let the brain know that they're under stress. As you continue to pull the Blu Tack at both ends then stress intensifies and therefore the response would intensify. If you kept pulling then eventually it would get so overstretched that a tear would begin to emerge and, by continuing to pull, this tear would get bigger and bigger until eventually the Blu Tack would snap. If you imagine the nerves during those final stages where the more it's being stretched the more stress is being put on to the nerves, then the nerves of our Blu Tack muscle would be telling the brain they're under even greater stress than earlier and that would be felt as more pain than earlier. The more the nerves are stretched the greater the pain response.

So, if the pain you're experiencing is the equivalent of an overstretched piece of Blu Tack, then hopefully you can see that by stretching it more (adding more stress to it) can often make things worse. If a muscle is already overstretched and under stress then stretching it more and adding more stress to it isn't the play. So, what is the solution? This brings us to the next key principle.

If something is overstretched, then something else is too short

Generally, muscles/ligaments/tendons don't just become overstretched by themselves. You know the score by now when I say that there are always exceptions. For example, I've had a couple of clients over the years that have torn a hamstring by slipping and doing the splits by accident. Acute, overstretching injuries do occur but for the vast majority of issues there is a functional imbalance that leads to an area becoming overstretched and painful. Our muscles, ligaments and tendons are all working together and trying to find that balance of optimal tension. If you think about the action of having a straight arm and then flexing at the elbow to bend your arm you can see how as numerous muscles have to fire and shorten to elevate your lower arm (e.g. the biceps) similarly many others will have to relax and lengthen to allow the movement to happen (e.g. the triceps). If all the muscles in your arm all tensed equally at the same time when your arm was straight then you wouldn't be able to bend your arm. That might seem very basic but it's important to visualise the relationships between areas of the body and different muscle groups and how these interlink for movements to occur. As one area shortens then another will lengthen but pain often occurs where an area is being asked to work in a lengthened, overstretched position too often. This will be a theme for most of the issues we'll cover. Before we move on however, we should cover the elephant in the room – if stretching an already overstretched muscle makes it worse, then why does it feel so nice to stretch it?

Stretching feels nice but make sure you're stretching the muscle that needs it

Psychologically and physically stretching feels nice, full stop. Normally the first thing we do in the morning is have a stretch out in bed. Stretching has numerous benefits including improved circulation; improved flexibility and range of movement; relaxation and stimulation of the release of endorphins. So, with all these benefits you can see why stretching feels so nice. But what the body doesn't do is tell you which part you should be stretching. If you stretch a short, tight muscle it feels nice. If you stretch an already lengthened, overstretched muscle it also feels nice. This is where the difficulty in knowing what to stretch comes in. If you are stretching an already overstretched muscle further you are probably doing more harm than good. This is why when someone calls me about an issue I'll often tell them not to stretch anything until we've had a look and worked out what's going on, as giving advice on stretching the wrong muscle could easily make the situation worse.

The main goal of this book is to get you to think about how your body is working and what areas may be under stress. I'm always telling clients that it's the muscles that don't hurt that you need to be thinking about. Here I have included a couple of examples to show you the principles in action before we move on to start looking at specific areas of the body.

Example one: sore hamstring in a football player

For this example I've picked a football player but this could relate to numerous other sports. A common client presentation might look like this:

> I've been feeling my right hamstring for a few weeks. It feels sore right in the middle of the muscle. I tried having a week off and it didn't really help and I've been stretching it more because it feels tighter but it still seems to be getting worse. What should I do?

Every client presentation is unique so to add some history to this example and to keep it simple we'll say that this is their first issue and their reason for seeking treatment. They've never had an injury before hamstring or otherwise. As this client is feeling the pain in the middle of the muscle it immediately resonates with the Blu Tack concept. The middle of the muscle is being overstretched through movement so something must be tight somewhere else. Through questioning we find out that this person is predominantly right-footed when they play. Think about the common actions involved in football –running, jumping, sprinting and kicking. For some of these actions the right leg will be used more. Next, thinking about mechanics, a lot of those movements are dynamic and explosive. To generate the power for many of these movements, especially kicking and sprinting, the quadriceps and hip flexor muscles on the front of the upper leg have a big part to play. Therefore, knowing that this person is predominantly right-footed when they play, we would likely find that although the right hamstring is the site of the pain (the symptom), it is in fact the quadriceps and hip flexors on the right being short and tight (the cause) that are causing the hamstring to be overstretched and painful.

I know I've invented this client but there are some key clues in the initial presentation which give hints as to the potential issue. Firstly, the pain is only in one leg suggesting there must be an imbalance somewhere. Secondly, rest didn't make any difference which makes sense because if one muscle group is short (quadriceps/hip flexors) and one overstretched (hamstrings) then rest alone won't make the short muscle any looser and when the person returns to activity as the same mechanical imbalance is present the pain is still felt. Thirdly, stretching it more was making it worse which would hint that the area being stretched may well be overstretched already.

Hopefully, you can see how this example fits in with the principles but here's a summary:

- **Pain is just the symptom.**
  Although the pain was in the right hamstring the hamstring itself wasn't the cause of the issue.
- **If it hurts don't stretch it.**
  As the hamstring was already overstretched then stretching it more would make it worse.
- **If something is overstretched then something else is too short.**
  In this scenario the quadriceps and hip flexors on the right leg were short and tight which then lead to the stress on the hamstring.
- **Stretching feels nice but make sure you're stretching the muscle that needs it.**
  This person felt they needed to stretch their hamstring even more as it was sore and it felt like it was the right thing to do, when in fact it would have been making things worse.

The advice for this client would probably involve lots of right hip flexor (and probably, although not definitely, quadricep) stretching and stopping hamstring stretching temporarily. However, I'm not suggesting that this is the solution to all hamstring pain. The hamstring may have become so overstretched that there may have been a small tear and a programme of strengthening may be required. The hip flexor may well be tight due to other reasons, not just football, so an exploration of other activities would be needed to ensure a comprehensive plan of action which would likely involve stretching and strengthening of a number of different areas. I know I keep referring to this but there is no 'one-size-fits-all' approach. However, hopefully you can see the importance of making sure the correct areas are being focussed on, worked on and changed and that, more often than not, the areas that actually need changing aren't asking for help. It will often take a bit of investigating and connecting of the dots to work out where the true source of the problem is.

Example two: Sore upper back when sat at a computer

For this example I'm going to pick someone working at a fixed desk on a computer with a single screen. As you can imagine there are a number of variations that could be applied here such as, the number of screens being used; whether it's a laptop, a computer, or a tablet; whether the desk is a sit to stand desk; whether the person hot desks etc. But this invented person works at the same desk every day with the same setup and the same chair and their story might sound a bit like this:

> I can't pinpoint the pain all the time but it feels like it's somewhere around my shoulder blade and sometimes goes up into my neck or into my shoulder. It's pretty bad on both sides but probably a bit worse on the right. I've had it on and off for months but it never really fully goes away. It usually gets worse as the day goes on at work and sometimes it's bad in the evening if I'm sat on the sofa. It feels like it's really stiff and tight and needs freeing up. I don't remember ever doing anything to it, like an injury or anything and can't really remember when it started. I think I just woke up with it one morning and it's stayed with me since. It was really bad when I woke up Monday so I thought 'I've had enough now' and I want to get it sorted.

As with the first example you're always looking for little clues. Does it hurt more on the right because they're right-handed? The fact that they don't remember specifically doing anything to hurt it suggests it could be from a cumulative process and as a result of a repetitive/ overuse issue. Comments like, "it's really stiff and tight and needs freeing up," might mean they've already been trying to stretch it and free it up already. If it were bad Monday morning then what had they been up to at the weekend that could have aggravated the underlying problem? These are the kinds of questions that you can ask yourself when trying to figure out what's causing you pain and why.

Through questioning this made-up person, it turns out they are right-handed. This has the potential to be a factor as the chances are that this side gets used more day-to-day compared to the left but it probably wouldn't be enough to just pin it all on that. Also, nothing significant has changed recently for this client (i.e. they haven't had a new bed, car, sofa or seat at work) so, again, there's not a single issue to pin it to. Where the neck and back had been sore for a few months they do disclose that they have started stretching the neck and upper back recently to try and 'free it up' but that this hasn't really helped. After initially saying they hadn't been up to much at the weekend it turns out they'd been doing a lot of gardening, mainly digging but didn't think that was really relevant as it didn't hurt any more than normal when they were doing it. Finally, upon digging deeper about their work station setup, it turns out that their screen is slightly off centre to the left, the person they speak to most is on their left and occasionally they have to reference books for their work which they would always have to their left as the mouse is on the right.

Again, I know this person is made-up but I've seen a lot of clients presenting with similar issues with similar causes over the years. It's a classic case of a cumulative process in action where a few consistent stresses on an area over a period of weeks and months can lead to a bigger issue in the end. In this instance, although the pain was being experienced through the neck and upper back, these muscles are the ones that are overstretched and irritated. If you think of looking left to chat to a friend then you'd be stretching the right-hand side. Having your screen just a little bit off centre won't do you any immediate harm but if you think about that multiplied by hundreds of hours at work then you can see how this could add to the irritation. If you think about the action of digging you'd be leaning forward and reaching out in front of you, again stretching the neck and upper back and more on the right-hand side being right-handed. When we sit on our sofas we tend to sink or slump into them so, again, this can round our shoulders and overstretch the neck and upper back. Put all of this together and you'd end up with short muscles through the chest and anterior (front) neck keeping quiet and not complaining and then the overstretched, grumpy muscles through the upper back and posterior (back) neck.

Here's a quick summary of how this example also fits in with the principles:

- **Pain is just the symptom.**
  Although the pain was in the upper back those muscles themselves weren't the cause of the issue.
- **If it hurts don't stretch it.**
  As the muscles of the upper back were already overstretched then stretching them more would make the situation worse.
- **If something is overstretched then something else is too short.**
  In this scenario the muscles of the chest and the anterior neck were short and tight which, through the rounding of the shoulders and pulling the head forward, then lead to the stress on the upper back and posterior neck muscles.
- **Stretching feels nice but make sure you're stretching the muscle that needs it.**
  This person felt they needed to stretch out their upper back even more as it felt stiff and restricted. In fact, trying to 'free up' the 'stiff' back would have created more stress on the area and made things more painful.

There are a few minor changes that this client could make that would make a significant difference when put together. Firstly, stopping stretching the back and neck would be key as these muscles are already overstretched. Some subtle changes at work, such as making sure the screen is exactly in the middle, getting into the habit of swivelling round on their chair if they want to chat to the person on their left and trying to use the mouse left-handed can all make a difference. Stretching out the short muscles, in this case primarily the chest muscles, would have a significant impact on reducing the stress on the upper back and neck. Also, in the evenings, instead of sitting or lying on the sofa for extended periods of time if this could be broken up with the occasional lying flat on your back on the floor this would really help with taking the stress off the upper back and neck.

I'm aware I've picked a couple of examples that do fit nicely into the principles but there really are so many others that I've come across over the years that also fit in that it can't all just be coincidence! If neither of the above examples have applied to you then I'm sure there will be other examples throughout this book that will resonate as I've tried to cover the most common scenarios that I come across.

We're now going to start looking at specific areas of the body, starting at the top and working our way down, so some of the issues in example two will feature as we look at the neck and upper back first. As I've alluded to many times already, discomfort normally arises from an imbalance in the network as a whole rather than from just a single point. So, when we look at sections in isolation, for example the neck and upper back, we'll often refer to other areas of the body that could also be linked. I'm always trying to get you to look at the bigger picture and the system as a whole rather than having tunnel vision on what hurts because if you focus too much on the symptom then it's easy to miss a potentially bigger, more important issue that could be the key to numerous other problems. As I've already mentioned a few times, you're never fixed, cured or injury-proof but if you can have the best understanding of how your body works and interacts with itself and its surroundings then I believe you can get the most out of yourself and enjoy a life with as little pain as possible.

CHAPTER 3

Neck and Upper Back

I regularly get asked, "What area do you treat the most?" and "What's the most common injury you treat?" When I first started out I don't remember a pattern to what I saw or who I treated and I would say that's still pretty much the case now. However, I think I would say now if I had to name a body area that I treat the most that it probably would be the upper back/neck. Only just but it probably has become the most frequently asked for area in treatment over the last few years. I can't pinpoint a single reason that would have caused this subtle change but, as per example two in the last chapter, I wonder if it is a case of cumulative effect in action. Most of us do have a selection of, or possibly all of, the following items – mobile phone, tablet, laptop, smart watch, games console, car. The use of these encourage us to look down more than up resulting in a slightly rounded posture and I wonder if the cumulative effect of years of using some or all of these items is leading to more people asking for help with the neck and upper back.

Clients will present with any number of issues relating to the neck and upper back. This area is often described as having twinged, spasmed or locked up. People often seek treatment due to headaches, both acute and chronic. I'll frequently hear that someone's neck feels 'stiff' or 'tight' and that it needs to be 'clicked' or 'freed up'. This isn't a conclusive list but most of us will have experienced one or more of these issues over our lifetime. In the vast majority of these cases the pain comes due to an imbalance of short/tight muscles pulling against tired/overstretched muscles. As always, the key is understanding which is which and what you can do to make a positive change to the situation.

With the neck and upper back muscles I usually like to start with a simple question, "How often do you look up throughout the day?" Of course, there are some activities where this has to be the case such as rock climbing or painting/plastering a ceiling. But for the vast majority of the population, over the course of a 24-hour period, how often do we look up? Conversely, what percentage of our day do we spend looking forward and maybe more importantly, how much time do we spend looking down? While thinking about this a few years ago a client chose the analogy of a bowling ball on the end of two fingers and I loved it. If your neck in this scenario is the two fingers and if your head, the bowling ball, was held neutrally all day long the muscles of the neck would be equally tired. But imagine tilting that bowling ball just a little bit forward and imagine how much harder the muscles in your fingers would have to work to stop the ball from dropping. With that in mind I want you to think about your head position in the following everyday activities:

- driving
- sleeping
- looking at your phone/tablet/smart watch
- sitting on the sofa
- taking part in your favourite exercise/sport.

In terms of trying to keep the balance between anterior and posterior muscles, some of the above activities can be more anterior dominant. When you're driving do you find yourself a bit round-shouldered with your head forward? Do you normally find yourself looking down at your phone? I'm not suggesting these things are bad for you but I'm just trying to get you to think about how your body is working throughout the day. If your favourite exercise is rock climbing then you have a better chance of having strong neck extensor muscles (muscles on the back of the neck) as you will be using them more to look up. However, I've had clients over the years try rock climbing and it's made their neck worse as those extensor muscles were too weak and ended up getting irritated. I'm not going to go through every sport one-by-one but I enjoy playing golf. I'm aware though that this requires lots of looking down with slightly rounded shoulders and also, being right-handed, a lot more looking left than right, as that's the way your head has to move through the swing (much like a right-handed batter in cricket). I don't believe golf and cricket are bad for you but they do ask different questions of your body than a more neutral activity such as swimming. But if you had a sore neck after golf, where you'd just done lots of looking down and twisting of the neck and shoulders, would stretching the neck out even more help? I think it would make it worse. After you've spent half an hour looking down at your phone and your upper back starts aching (think about how heavy that bowling ball is to hold up) is it good to stretch the upper back out even more or would it be better to spend five minutes lying flat on your back on the floor to give those muscles a break? If we can keep ourselves as upright and neutral for as much of the day as possible then our muscles won't get as fatigued and irritated and therefore, from both a pain and recovery perspective, we would have a better chance of getting higher quality sleep in a better position and have the best chance of feeling good the next day. This is a big challenge as for most of us our jobs, activities, exercises and sports don't encourage us to have a neutral posture. Therefore, if we can understand as much as possible about how our bodies work day-to-day, we have the best chance to keep them working at their best.

Without oversimplifying it, the biggest challenge for the neck and upper back muscles is the battle of front (anterior) versus back (posterior). As discussed previously, the majority of activities and actions we undertake encourage us to look down more than up and have our arms in front of us rather than behind us. Throw in the influence of gravity as well and it's easy to see how the anterior muscles can shorten up and how the posterior muscles can become overstretched. I find that visualising it like a see-saw helps. If you had two people of equal size, one person on either side of the see-saw, then it would remain level as the stresses/tension on the see-saw would be equal. If you added an extra person to one side of the see-saw then that side would go down and the other side would go up. It's a simple way of looking at it but as one side of the see-saw compresses down towards the ground the other side extends away from it. Many muscles within the body are working in synergy with each other and in many cases as one muscle group shortens then the other muscle group will lengthen (remember the bicep and tricep example from earlier). More often than not it will be the overstretched muscle that is under stress and experiencing the pain but the key is to then find the short, tight muscle/muscles that are causing this stress. As well as the battle of anterior versus posterior, we have the challenge of balancing left versus right. Many of the examples and activities we cover throughout this book will have elements of both challenges involved.

If you've had treatment before, or have ever looked into neck and back pain yourself, you may have come across the phrases anterior chain and posterior chain. If not, don't worry as it's pretty simple to explain. It ties in nicely with the front versus back challenge we referred to above. Imagine you're standing side on and you drew a line from the top of your head down to your feet that split your body in half, dividing it in to front and back (if you want to look into it a bit more it's called the coronal or frontal plane). The muscles, ligaments and tendons in front of the dividing line make up the anterior chain and those behind the dividing line make up the posterior chain. Simple.

So, with the neck it's often a case of the anterior chain muscles (neck flexors) versus the posterior chain muscles (neck extensors) and with the upper back it's often the anterior chain (neck flexors, chest, biceps) versus the posterior chain (neck extensors, upper back, triceps).

Below are a couple of illustrations of the neck and upper torso that show you some of the most common muscles that I have to work on. It's important to note here that while every muscle, ligament and tendon in the body is important and has a significant role to play I feel it would be a little overwhelming to name every single part here so I must stress I'm picking the ones that I feel are most significantly involved in the most common issues I see. It won't be an all-encompassing list of every muscle in the neck and torso but hopefully it will show you enough detail and allow you to use it as a reference point for both the future and also for now as you're reading this.

Common challenges

We've already alluded to this but we can generalise a lot of the common challenges in the neck and upper back under the umbrella

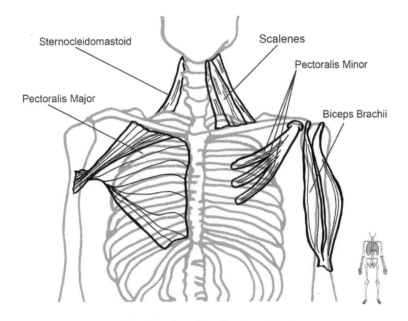

Image 1 – anterior neck and torso

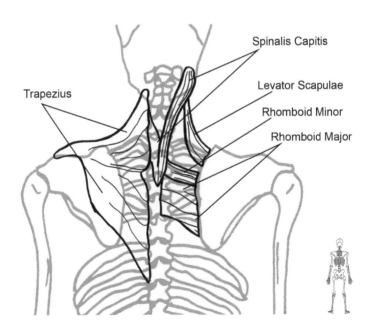

Image 2 – posterior neck and torso

of anterior chain versus posterior chain. This isn't an all-encompassing list and many have already been mentioned but below, in no particular order I must add, are the most common causes (not symptoms) of neck and upper back pain that I see:

- driving
- looking at your phone/tablet/smart watch
- working at a desk
- sitting on the sofa
- some exercises/sports (especially those where you're predominantly right or left-handed)
- stress
- looking after a new born baby
- gardening/DIY
- reading
- sleeping

Now, we'll work our way through this list and see what muscles and actions generally lead to this discomfort. We'll then end this section by discussing what we can do about these issues. There will be little tips along the way for each activity but at the end we'll cover the most effective stretches and preventative measures you can take to reduce the stress on your body from these activities. (The tips will be ideas to try, not definitive rules, so whenever you try something different make sure you feel confident and safe in doing so.)

Driving

It doesn't just have to be long distance driving that leads to discomfort. For many people just a 10-minute trip can be enough for things to kick off, whether that's a general ache in the muscles or a twinge when they look over their shoulder. There is a correlation between the length of time you're driving and the stress on your neck and upper back. If you are more tense than normal before the drive or if the drive itself is more intense than normal (severe weather, lots of traffic, other people driving badly) then this is bound to contribute as well. Driving is a classic example of an activity where your arms are out in front of you and it's easy for your head to be further forward than it needs to be. Our arms are usually also slightly bent when we drive rather than locked out straight. There's not going to be a situation where your arms are reaching out behind you and you look up and back to counteract the driving position. So, with all this in mind, it's very common for the pectoralis muscles (pecs) and biceps to tighten up through driving. This in turn lengthens the rhomboids and mid/lower trapezius muscles (traps) and many people complain of an aching between their shoulder blades when driving. If the head is being pulled forward a little through driving then this occurs due to the flexors shortening up and therefore stretching the extensors. As a result the discomfort is often felt through the back of the neck, be that aching, twinges, spasms, headaches etc. Just a reminder that after we've looked at each activity individually we'll then discuss the best stretches to do and those to avoid.

Tips:

- Try having your seat a little more upright, ideally almost at 90 degrees, so that the seat supports your upper back. Many people lean forward away from their seat which puts more stress on their upper back.
- Make sure your rear-view mirror is set up correctly so that it encourages you to sit more upright in the seat. If you gradually slump when you're driving, which is very common and often goes unnoticed, when you check the rear-view mirror you'll see some of the roof lining which will remind you to sit up taller.
- Keep an eye on whether you lean on your arm rest or center console when you're sat in traffic or going along the motorway. If you're leaning down on one side then your neck will have to counteract that lean to make your head level for driving which will lead to shortening/lengthening of the muscles.

Looking at your phone/tablet/smart watch

What makes this extra tricky is that in the modern world we probably look at our devices more than we think we do, sometimes maybe even without consciously noticing we're doing it. Looking at our devices can cause irritation whether it be in the form of prolonged looking at a screen, the cumulative effect of repetitive looking for short periods of time or a combination of the two. The key to this is how we use the devices. How often do we look at these with our head in a neutral position? More often than not it involves us looking down, ranging from slightly looking down to sat on the sofa looking down at a screen on your lap. Anatomically, the pattern of anterior shortening can easily be repeated here. The neck flexors shorten up as we look down at our device and the pecs and biceps will shorten as the device is held in front of us. Therefore, the usual suspects of the posterior chain are put under excess stress. However, we also have the challenge of keeping a neutral head position in terms of side-to-side, left versus right, not just front and back. Do we look one way more than the other when using our devices? Are we therefore potentially stretching one side more than the other?

Tips:

- If you know you're going to be looking at a screen for a while try to position the screen so it is elevated or supported so that your head would be in a neutral position.
- Make sure that you are looking square on to your screen.
- If you're right-handed check whether you always look down and to the right to look at your phone/watch. If so try and use your phone/watch with your left hand some of the time to try and balance up.
- Try using your phone while lying flat on your back on the floor. This can encourage the head to be in a more relaxed and neutral position. However, holding your device out in front of you in this position comes with its own dangers (especially if you're tired and not fully concentrating and drop your phone on your face like I've done before) so please be careful!

Working at a desk

Desk working really highlights the postural challenges of anterior versus posterior and left versus right. There are so many scenarios where we can find ourselves more round-shouldered than optimal, looking down more than we'd like and looking one way more than the other. We've already covered many of the contributing factors in example two in the last chapter but we can add a couple more here. Nowadays, lots of clients say they have to work with two or more screens and this brings another challenge to the table. It's unlikely that, in the event of using two screens, that the screen time will be split exactly 50/50 between the two screens. There will also inevitably be times where the upper body might be facing one way and the neck another. That in itself isn't that big an issue but if those same movements are repeated, e.g. regularly typing on the screen on the right while regularly turning to look at the screen on the left, then an imbalance will eventually occur between the muscles on the left and right which could create discomfort. Again, it would be rare to be looking up or to have your arms behind your back while at a desk so it's reasonable to expect the anterior chain tightness and the posterior chain to be overstretched.

Tips:

- If you have more than one screen and you use one more than the other/others, try swapping your screens around at lunchtime or day-by-day to make sure you're not always using the same muscles in the same way.
- Put an alert/reminder/alarm on your screen so that you regularly get up and away from your desk to ensure you don't get stuck in a position for too long.
- If you're in a position where you know you're out of balance, e.g. you only ever look forward or left at work because you're at the end of the desk and there's only a wall to your right, change where you sit so you're more balanced.
- Get a sit to stand/adjustable desk so that you can alternate your position throughout the day.

Sitting on the sofa

This is a tricky one as the sofa is one of those places that we go to relax and unwind which is essential for the maintenance of a decent work/life balance. However, with the intentions being to relax and unwind, we can find ourselves staying in a certain position for an extended period of time. That's fine if that position is good but quite often this isn't the case. We might be lying on our sides with our neck twisted to see the television, or lying resting on the arm rest, or with our legs tucked up underneath us or looking down at a screen of one of our devices. The list goes on. In isolation for a brief period of time, looking at your phone on the sofa isn't going to cause you any significant issues. However, if you always sit the same way or in the same spot on the sofa, maybe looking at your phone and then looking left or right up at the television back to your phone, this repetition, over a period of weeks, months and years could lead to muscle imbalances and eventually pain.

Most sofas encourage us to slump into them which again encourages rounding of the shoulders and then further overstretching of the upper back and posterior chain. We are unlikely to be looking up at a screen while on the sofa so the potential is there again for anterior shortening and posterior lengthening with the muscles of the neck.

Tips:

- Try mixing up where you sit on the sofa so you don't get stuck in the same position.
- Make sure that your head and neck are neutral (not looking one way more than the other) when watching television or looking at a screen. You may need to relocate the television or sofa for this to work.
- Try not to lie with your head on the arm rest as if you're lying on your back this flexes your neck a lot and if you're lying on your side it often stretches one side more than the other.

Some exercises/sports (especially those where you're predominantly right or left-handed)

Sports and exercise are essential to health but many do have postural challenges. As we're looking at the upper body here then we'll focus on sports/exercises that are more relevant to these areas but, as always, the list won't include every sport. We covered golf a little earlier in the chapter but any sport that encourages or requires you to be more right or left-handed has the potential to create imbalance. This pretty much covers any racket or bat sport, or any sport where throwing is involved as the vast majority of us do have a dominant or preferred hand to throw or hit with. Most combat sports encourage you to have a stance that isn't square on so rotation and therefore imbalances are inevitable. Even with activities where we are square on and neutral, such as cycling or running, gravity does encourage us to lean forward a little which can then have an impact on the upper back. Also, the head position in cycling is different to most activities we do day-to-day. Swimming can create imbalances if you regularly do one stroke more than the others, or if when you're doing front crawl you always breathe on the same side meaning you only ever twist your neck one way.

Strengthening wise balance is key. If you are slightly anterior dominant (which as we've already shown through the previous examples is more probable than not) then going to the gym and doing lots of chest and bicep strengthening will likely only add to the imbalance between anterior and posterior. Doing activities such as shoulder press or pull-ups are great if everything is neutral but if one shoulder sits further forward than the other because it's your dominant side then you may find that doing pull-ups actually highlights the imbalance and that they're not done equally or that they cause discomfort. Where so much of this is about balance it's important to highlight that I'm not just going through and pointing out all the issues with every sport and exercise. I just want you to think about how your body works during these activities and then what you need to do to stretch and strengthen accordingly to make sure you get the full benefits from doing these activities rather than picking up injuries.

Tips:

- Consider whether any activity you do could be made more neutral. For example, maybe you could teach yourself to breathe both sides when swimming.
- Try to make sure any activities you do aren't exaggerating an imbalance further.

Stress

I said sofas were a tricky one but this could be the trickiest of them all. It's an unrealistic target to aim for zero stress but it is obvious that the more stress we have the more tension we carry. The reason for mentioning it is that if we have imbalances then stress tends to exacerbate these imbalances. It's hard to blame stress directly for issues but it does play a significant part. If we are tense we tend to be a little more round-shouldered, which yet again feeds into the anterior versus posterior challenge.

Tips:

- This doesn't really need saying but the less stress the better for your physical health.
- Try breaking up your day with periods of lying flat on your back on the floor for a few minutes.
- Try activities that help to regulate your body and breathing such as meditation.

Looking after a new born baby

This might seem a strange one at first but once again it focuses on the challenge of anterior versus posterior. Be it feeding the baby, changing nappies, playing with the baby, looking at the baby or carrying the baby, all these activities involve us rounding our shoulders and looking down. This is not an attempt to warn people off having children or to take any of the joy away but I get so many new clients (both male and female) who come in with new neck/back pains that have recently had a new born baby and, although not the only factor, it's often one of the more significant factors in their discomfort. However, as with all the other examples, if you have that awareness of how you are using your body then you can do the right activities to counteract these challenges.

Tips:

- If you are expecting a baby then, for both parents, it's worth trying to make yourself as strong and upright as you can beforehand as these postural challenges are going to happen (we'll cover strengthening ideas later in the chapter).
- If possible and for as long as you feel confident in doing so, try not to hold the baby on the same side all the time.

Gardening/DIY

Gardening and/or DIY are often responsible for lots of issues and discomfort. The most common scenario (like example two in the last chapter) is that a client will suffer a few days after the activity and won't connect the two together. Saying that, there have been a few occasions over the years where a client's neck has gone into spasm while painting or they've tweaked a muscle in their upper back while digging. But, more often than not, it's the delayed reaction a few days later that catches people out. There aren't many activities in the garden or in DIY projects that require you to have your arms behind your back and to look up. It's more likely that you'll find yourself in positions where you're kneeling down over flowerbeds, digging, sanding down a door frame or trimming a hedge. These activities usually require you to have your hands out in front of you for extended periods of time, sometimes holding something heavy, usually looking down more than up and often doing a repetitive movement. Again, doing a single action for a brief period of time is unlikely to cause an issue but if you start an activity in the morning and suddenly you find out you're hungry and it's mid-afternoon and you've been painting for six hours, issues can occur. I'm sure you've guessed it by now but most activities involved in gardening and/or DIY are anterior dominant and put stress on the posterior chain.

Tips:

- Taking regular breaks is essential to break up repetitive activities and reduce the risk of overuse issues.
- If you can and please be careful with this, you could try using your less dominant hand more often rather than just using one side all day. (With something like sanding or painting this isn't too dangerous but be careful if you want to try something like digging with your less dominant side.)
- Think about whether your body is strong enough for the activity. For example, consider whether your body wants you to be balancing on top of a ladder and reaching out in front of you with a hedge trimmer trying to carefully trim the top of the hedge.

Reading

Now I wouldn't class reading as an extreme sport but you'd be surprised how many people get issues from a seemingly simple activity. Primarily, like in a lot of activities, we do tend to look down when we're reading. Also, it's easy to find yourself sat in the same position for a long time especially if it's a good book. As you're reading this right now pause and think about the position you're in. The chances are you'll be looking down slightly but also is your head neutral? Are you reading looking towards one side over the other? This might not seem important but if you usually tend to tilt your head the same way when you read in bed or on the sofa then the repetitive nature of this activity could lead to stress on the area over time. Countless clients, even with pre-warning of the 'dangers' of reading will come back from holidays with neck and/or upper back pain with reading often being the primary cause of the discomfort. Once again, the potential is there with reading for anterior shortening and posterior lengthening.

Tips:

- If you always hold your book in the same hand then try alternating hands to make sure your neck has a better chance of being balanced.
- If you know you're going to be reading for a while you could try putting your book onto a stand and have it set at eye level so you don't have to hold the book and look down.
- Like many other activities, try to have regular breaks to ensure you're not sat in the same position for a prolonged period of time.

<u>Sleeping</u>

It's hard to say sleeping is a cause of neck and upper back pain but similarly it can't be ignored as a factor. On rare occasions you can point the finger at the sleeping position itself but so often I hear, "I've probably just slept funny" as the reason for pain when this is rarely the case. With a small number of clients, changing their head or shoulder position when they sleep has done the trick over time. But, more often than not, your sleep position is determined by how your body functions during your waking hours. Sleeping may well highlight the underlying issues but it is rarely the cause. This is good news because it's much easier said than done to just change how you sleep. If you sleep on your front looking the same way all night you will put stress on your neck. If you spent eight hours of your day looking left you'd expect a reaction so, although when you're asleep there's less stress on your body, it still wouldn't be ideal. But say your job requires you to look left more than right all day then is it purely a coincidence that you sleep looking to the left or does that play a factor? Without oversimplifying it, if you go to bed wonky you're not suddenly going to wake up perfect in the morning. Many people have pain at night because, although their body is resting, it's not resting in a good position so rest can sometimes highlight your imbalances and issues further. Another possible contributor to imbalance could be your pillows. Again, it might sound obvious but we're always looking for as neutral position as possible for the neck and upper back so if you sleep on your side then you want to have your head in a level position. Pillows come in all shapes and sizes so there isn't a rule here but it may be the case that if you sleep with one pillow your head isn't being supported enough and is tilting down towards the mattress. Likewise, if you have three pillows then you could possibly be tilting your neck too far the other way and not be in a neutral position. You can spend a fortune on pillows that sell themselves as the miracle cure as they essentially mould around your neck to give you the perfect individual support. In theory that's great if your neck is neutral and balanced in the first place but if you are out of balance then all you end up doing is spending a lot of money for a product that reinforces your incorrect position. I've had a few clients who have bought these pillows when they were out of balance and it made their symptoms worse. My advice is always to try and make your body the best it can be instead of spending money on things that claim they can do that for you.

Tips:

- There's lots of conflicting information about the 'best sleeping position' so don't overthink it.
- It's hard to change how you sleep but it's easier to get your body more efficient and neutral during the day by doing activities that you can control, which in turn gives you a better chance of sleeping in a better position.
- If you sleep on your side make sure you have your pillow/pillows so that your neck is level when you sleep.

Whiplash

There is a lot of misinformation and confusion around whiplash and this is often down to the insurance companies. I was in a small car accident a few years ago and, although I repeatedly told my insurance company I was completely fine, they kept trying to convince me that I would get whiplash symptoms eventually. I was told that if I had any neck discomfort at all or headaches at any point over the following six months I should ring up and make a claim for whiplash. It's ridiculous and it can lead to a stigma around whiplash where 'it's not a real thing' and people just say they've got it to get a pay-out. There isn't a 'set in stone' rule but generally the severity of the whiplash symptoms is linked to the severity of the accident. However, this is not a guarantee. Symptoms can take a few days to show (I'm not sure about six months later though!) and it's often described like a clamp or a vice that's tightening slowly as the muscles gradually tense up and go into 'protection mode'. Physiologically it's very clever, much like when you twist your ankle and swelling occurs to make the joint stiff and less mobile for self-preservation. As clever as it is if you have ever experienced whiplash symptoms you will know how restrictive and uncomfortable it can be.

Whiplash in the neck occurs when the neck is forcefully hyperflexed and then hyperextended (or vice versa). We know the most common cause of this is car accidents but it can easily happen in contact sports (football, rugby, boxing etc.) as well as in a fall. Due to the variety of ways you can get whiplash and the different degrees of severity it's hard to give specific timeframes on recovery. The severity of the symptoms is often linked to the severity of the accident. I've had clients with minor issues where it takes a few weeks to return to normal. Most, more severe issues can take a few months but I've had some clients, in very severe accidents, where it's taken upwards of three years to return to normal. The best way I can think to describe it is to imagine that there's a window of activities that the body is happy to do when everything is working well. If we get fitter or stronger then we become capable of doing more activities so our window expands. When you get whiplash that window shrinks and even small, simple actions are perceived as 'too much' by the brain. Your body becomes more tentative and is worried about you hurting yourself and causing further damage. As we said symptoms can often take a few days to develop. Most people may feel a little shook up but generally ok initially but then the pain takes hold over the coming days.

The key to the quickest recovery is to not be too immobile for too long while, at the same time, respecting that you are in pain and the body is in protection mode and your window of comfortable activities has reduced significantly. If there was a way to know how much and how quickly to push yourself with getting back to normal that would be ideal but unfortunately that doesn't exist. You have to gradually try to expand your window of activities by carefully trying to improve mobility and when we say mobility, it doesn't mean forcefully stretching or rolling your neck. Remember that the neck has just gone through a massively stressful experience where it has been maximally stretched in one direction and then another, so if you start stretching it again this is only likely to add more stress. Returning back to your window, gradual improvement is the key here and no doubt, along the way, you will overdo it at times and the body will let you know and you'll feel as though you've taken a step back. But without attempting to take steps forward in the first place your recovery can last a lot longer than it needs to. As I say to everyone you will never know if you could have done more but you'll always find out when you've done too much. Of course, I'm biased here but I think hands-on treatment is essential to help 'turn down' the muscles, as clients will often describe it as if the muscles are fully switched on and turned up to the maximum. Treatment can only be light initially but every little helps in terms of encouraging the muscles to relax and allow gentle increases in movement. Again, at times you'll get disheartened when you accidentally overdo it but the longer you leave it the harder it is to convince the muscles to let go and return to how they used to be. In some cases this can be a process that takes years but, over time, you can usually regain full movement, strength and, maybe more importantly, confidence and eventually get back to where you were before your whiplash injury.

Bulging, herniated and slipped discs

These diagnoses are often interchangeable depending on the professional you see but essentially they're all giving you loosely the same information. Our vertebral discs act like cushions between each of the vertebrae in our spine. The discs themselves consist of softer cartilage in the middle with a surrounding layer of tougher cartilage. For this reason they are often described as little jam doughnuts between your vertebrae. Like everything else in the body these discs are subject to wear and tear due to the stresses and strains we put our bodies through on a daily basis. We'll discuss this in further detail in the next section but over time the discs gradually become dehydrated and, as a result, become stiffer which can cause the outer layer to start bulging out. Keeping to the food analogies it's sometimes described like a hamburger that's too big for its bun or a jam doughnut where the jam has been squeezed out. Either way, this thickening and resulting protrusion of the outer layer of the disc *can* irritate the surrounding nerves and cause discomfort.

However, the emphasis is most definitely on the word *can* here. Imaging scans can tell you if there is any bulging or herniation but they can't guarantee that this is the cause of your pain. You can have a bulging disc and have no neck pain. Likewise, you can have neck pain and completely happy discs. I personally think that the way it is framed sometimes can have a massively detrimental effect on the person. Clients are rarely given potential solutions to the problem and are instead often given all sorts of conflicting information such as,

It's something you'll just have to live with.
It'll probably get better by itself.
It may never get better.

I want us to go back to the food analogies again. If you can visualise looking at the spinal column from behind you would ideally want the vertebrae to be stacked nicely on top of each other in a straight line from top to bottom (if you were looking from a side on view you'd want to see some curvature in the spine so that's why we're looking at it from behind in this analogy). So, we're looking at a lovely neutral spine and looking at the discs between the vertebrae and we can see that, as they are stacked up perfectly on top of each other, it wouldn't matter how much jam was in the doughnut or how big the hamburger was because if they're perfectly stacked there's no bulging. However, let's put a skull on top of this spinal column and have it tilting down to the left-hand side slightly. How do you think that would affect the alignment of the vertebrae? By adding the force of the weight of the skull to the left-hand side, the vertebrae of the neck would no longer be stacked up perfectly on top of each other and the spinal column would bend slightly. So, imagine you're pinching down on the left side of the burger bun can you visualise the hamburger having to be forced across to the right slightly? You could almost say it was 'slipping' to the right. In theory, if it slipped enough it could eventually push against a nearby nerve and pain would be the result (and there you have your slipped disc). But this pain has occurred as a reaction to the forces being felt more on one side over the other side. When the spinal column is neutral then the forces are equal, the discs are aligned and, as such, nerve irritation is unlikely.

This point in itself also highlights a potential loophole with the imaging scans. When having a scan you are usually put into a neutral position with everything lined up perfectly for the scan. Realistically, if your issue is caused by functional misalignment when your body is being used, which is the most probable cause, then when you're put into a neutral position everything will look fine as it's in position A and isn't a reflection of the positions you're in when the pain strikes. Likewise, this is often why lying flat on your back on the floor relieves symptoms because you are overriding the normal stresses of alignment and gravity and getting them to work in your favour. In recent times some facilities have started scanning people stood up and this is a massive step forward as it can give a truer reflection of how the body is being used. However, this is probably more relevant to lower backs so we'll cover that more in the next chapter.

Degenerative disc disease/spinal discopathy

We touched on this earlier but I wanted to give this its own little section. One of the biggest issues I face is getting people to trust their bodies again after diagnoses. As I'm working on this section, right on cue, I have just started seeing *another* client who has been 'diagnosed' with spinal discopathy after a scan following three months of headaches. She was understandably distressed with the diagnosis and was concerned for the future. I asked her what 'prognosis' she'd been given. What was the treatment plan? How had she been told to manage it? Her response was, unfortunately, as expected. She was told it was something she'd just have to live with and it would probably get worse as time went by. As for treatment, they were just going to carry on doing the same thing and hope it improved. How are you meant to feel hearing that news? It's basically like being told, "You've got a condition and there's nothing that can be done for you. All the best."

Day-by-day we add more wear and tear to our bodies. It's simple maths. A car with 100,000 miles on the clock has more wear and tear than a car that's done 1,000 miles and that's the way it is. Our discs will wear down and lose hydration the older we get. It's unavoidable. You could scan all the adults in the world and I'm sure the vast majority would be classed as having 'degenerative disc disease'. I find the words 'degenerative' and 'disease' so powerful for what is essentially natural wear and tear that we will all go through the more miles we put on the clock. When people are told they have a disease their response isn't usually a positive one so this causes so much unnecessary stress to them.

So, what's the cure for this 'disease' that isn't actually a disease? It all comes back to our old friend alignment. Think back to the last section – if the vertebrae are stacked up nicely on top of each other and under as equal stress as possible then you greatly reduce the risk of the discs being a significant factor altogether. At the time of writing I have seen the client I was referring to above for three sessions. Her job requires her to look down and to her left a lot more than any other position throughout the day. As such, in treatment so far, I have just worked on trying to lengthen the anterior muscles of her neck on the left (as they are short and tight) and help settle down the posterior muscles on the right (as they are overstretched and irritated). We've made sure she isn't stretching her neck at all and we're getting her to lie flat on her back for short periods as a way of giving the neck a break (unfortunately she can't do this at work but that would have been even more beneficial). When I saw her last week for her third session she said she's feeling loads better and hadn't had any headaches between sessions which was the first time in three months. We've got more work to do to get her even closer to neutral but it's a start and, considering that a few weeks ago she was told she had a disease and nothing could be done about it, she's in a much better place psychologically as well as physically. I wish I could say that her scenario was rare but it's not. This is a generalisation I know but there is often far too much emphasis put on investigations to discover diagnoses when the time could be better spent on making sure that your body is working at its most efficient and seeing whether you can get yourself out of pain by trying to get all your muscles working together to improve alignment.

General Tips

As I keep saying I can't cover every conceivable activity here but I'm sure you can see there are regular themes running through the list of the most common causes of neck and upper back pain. The challenge of balancing anterior versus posterior is consistent throughout but there are also some similarities between the tips for the different activities. The suggested tips are ideas that you might want to try and may include some you have already thought of and tried yourself but these tips can transcend into other activities as well.

A common thread to these tips is trying to do activities with your less dominant side. I'm trying to get you to think, "Do I need to do this activity with my stronger hand?" We've already listed a lot of activities above (such as using your phone or gardening) that you could try doing with your less dominant hand but we could easily include brushing your teeth, using the TV remote, drinking, knitting, sewing, doing puzzles, cooking, cleaning, bathing and showering to name but a few. The list is endless. You might think it's being a bit over the top but if you work out over your lifetime how many hours you are going to spend doing just one of these activities and if you only ever do these with one hand then the cumulative effect of this is going to cause a lot more stress to one side of the body than the other. For example, if you followed the recommended advice of brushing your teeth for two minutes in the morning and two minutes in the evening the average person would spend a total of 79 days or 1,896 hours over their lifetime brushing. Does that need to always be done with the same hand?

Another common thread is taking regular breaks and not doing repetitive activities for too long. Just to clarify a repetitive activity doesn't have to be a strenuous activity. As with sitting on the sofa or reading a book, being in the incorrect position for an extended period of time will eventually have consequences. You don't have to be moving for a position to cause stress on your body.

Now, in terms of stretching and strengthening, I am going to suggest some dos and don'ts. These are not set in stone and if you are in any doubt as to whether you should be doing any of these activities then, as always, please seek professional advice before attempting them. This is not an exhaustive list of all 'good' and 'bad' upper body stretches and strengthening exercises but this is my opinion based on my experiences as a therapist and a human. We'll start with the don'ts first and the chances are you will have done some, if not all, of these at one point or another. If you have that's ok but hopefully now it'll make sense why doing them probably hasn't really helped before.

What not to do

The idea of stretching and strengthening is to improve an issue, not make it worse. That might seem like the most obvious sentence in the world but so often you can end up doing stretches that make issues worse. Where most of the challenges arise from anterior shortening and posterior lengthening, stretching an already lengthened muscle further is going to make things worse. Therefore, I always advise people to avoid neck and upper back stretching. Stretching your neck and upper back more makes things worse. This contradicts a lot of advice but I feel strongly about this. To date, not just the majority but **every client** that has needed to stop neck and upper back stretching has improved and not gone back to it since. That might seem a bold claim but it's true and it works. By stopping stretching the neck and back you stop adding more stress to the area. This, combined with the correct stretches of the anterior chain is what makes the difference and leads you to having a pain-free neck and upper back.

In terms of strengthening where the anterior chain is often too dominant already, I try and advise clients to avoid doing activities that are likely to reinforce the imbalance. This often looks like avoiding activities such as chest and bicep strengthening and sit ups as these encourage even more rounding of the neck and shoulders.

What to do

So, now we know the incorrect activities let's think about what the correct ones are. For me, the number one upper body stretch is chest stretching. This massively helps to open out the anterior chain and immediately takes stress off the posterior chain. If you are in pain, though, then often clients will find lying flat on their back on the floor helps to 'switch off' some of the pain. Depending on the severity of the pain you may need a small towel rolled up underneath your neck as resting your head on the floor maybe too much of a push initially. An important side note here though is when you go to get up from lying on your back don't just sit up as that action shortens all the anterior chain. If possible try and roll round on to your side and on to all fours and get up that way. Another way of soothing the posterior chain (aside from getting treatment) is to use a tennis ball, rubber ball, spikey ball or foam roller on the muscles of the upper back to help clear out some of the fatigue and stress through those muscles.

In terms of strengthening upper back strengthening is massively important. If clients want to do chest strengthening as well then it's recommended that they train with a ratio of 3:1 back to chest. In short, train your upper back three times as much as your chest. The same ratio can be applied to tricep and bicep strengthening whereby you do three times as much on the triceps (posterior chain). To be honest most of us use our chest and biceps enough during the day so I'm happy if most of my clients don't train their chest or biceps at all but it's a personal choice.

Other factors

As alluded to earlier, this is not a conclusive list of all possible neck and upper back issues. There can be issues that are neurological in nature. Similarly, issues such as bone spurs or damaged vertebrae can also be factors. However, just because you have these issues doesn't mean that improvements can't still be made. I've had numerous clients who've been told they have bone spurs in their neck and will always have pain but we've still been able to get them out of pain by making their neck more neutral and reducing the stress on the vertebrae. Just because you've been told you have a condition or injury doesn't mean that it has to always be a problem for you.

CHAPTER 4

Shoulders

Shoulders are fascinating due to the complexity of the ranges of movement and functions they can undertake. From reaching down to pick something up off the floor, throwing something, reaching up to put something in a cupboard, reaching around behind you to put your coat on and everything in between, shoulders are amazing. However, having the capabilities to function in all these different ways brings with it the challenge of maintaining the strength, stability and flexibility required to do all these actions. Furthermore, we are constantly trying to achieve that balance while again facing the anterior versus posterior challenge and dealing with the fact that nearly all of us have a more dominant hand. If we used both shoulders equally throughout the day the first challenge of anterior versus posterior would still exist but the reality is that nearly all of us will, on top of that challenge, then be using one shoulder more than the other every day. If you've been unlucky enough to significantly injure your dominant side and had to ask your other side to step up then you may well be aware of how surprisingly difficult it can be to have full control of the less dominant side. I often hear phrases such as 'that arm's just for show' or 'it feels like it's wired up differently' or 'it's like someone else is controlling it'. Although it's definitely possible to train up your less dominant side (as hinted at in the general tips section of the last chapter) it's realistic to assume that over your lifetime one side will get used more than the other. As always, that fact in itself isn't a massive issue but having that awareness and appreciation for how your body functions is essential in potentially reducing your risk of pain and injuries and getting the most out of your body.

As with any area of the body the issues and pains associated with the shoulder can range from acute to chronic. Some acute issues may need immediate attention, such as dislocations and fractures, whereas the more chronic issues require attention over a longer period of time. As a soft tissue therapist I tend to see more chronic issues and more often than not these issues don't have a single initial cause. Shoulder issues frequently 'build up over time' or 'sneak in and gradually get worse'. Most clients won't remember doing anything in particular and the issue usually starts out as sporadic and a bit annoying and then builds up to becoming more of a consistent pain. It's also common that clients will feel that their shoulder 'pinches' or 'catches' and that they get pain shooting down the arm.

As per the last chapter, we're not going to go through every single muscle that can affect shoulder stability and functionality because we could have a whole book just on the shoulder. I'm choosing to cover the muscles that are associated with the most frequent issues and complaints that I come across with my clients. The most common issues usually involve anterior chain shortening of muscles such as the biceps and pecs, which then leads to stress in the posterior muscles such as the rotator cuff muscles as well as stress on the shoulder joint itself. If the joint is regularly being pulled forward and down then the compounding effect of this is usually a significant factor in contributing to irritation and pain. Frequently, rotator cuff inflammation can account for the pains that shoot/refer down the arm. Pain felt at the front or top of the shoulder is often due to the shoulder being more anteriorly rotated from being pulled forward by the tight anterior muscles. If the head of the humerus is sitting too far forward then there is inevitably stress on all the muscles around the shoulder as they work on trying to allow the shoulder to still function as well as possible while being in an incorrect position and out of balance.

Where we can take the shoulders through such a wide range of movements it's essential that we're doing this from the best starting position as possible. If the joint isn't in a great starting position before you reach up into the cupboard to grab something then when you do extend and rotate out to grab that cup then that 'extra' stress can often be a tipping point for discomfort to be felt. I try to explain to clients that when the shoulder isn't in an optimal position that it's like you're already starting one–zero down before you've even moved. The biggest challenge though, as is often the case in other areas of the body, is that we don't usually know that we're one–zero down in the first place until we feel pain. There is often no warning that the shoulder has reached its tipping point until we feel pain. I always say to clients that it would be great if a buzzer could go off telling us something's not quite right before we did an action that caused us pain but unfortunately the reality is we just experience pain and then have to try and work out what just happened and why it hurts.

This investigative challenge can occasionally be a simple one. Ask anyone who has ever dislocated their shoulder and it usually won't take long figuring out when it may have occurred. Trying to work out why you get searing pain in your shoulder first thing in the morning when trying to take your arm down from above your head in bed can be a trickier one to work out. Likewise, how can your shoulder be fine when lifting something heavy into your car but then you get an intense pain down the top of your arm when you reach up to shut the boot or reach out to grab the car keys off the kitchen worktop? I will often try and describe it to clients that when the shoulder isn't in an optimal position that it doesn't like surprises. So, using that last example about the car, if you prepare yourself to lift something heavy you are more likely to engage all the supporting muscles so the joint has a better chance of being stabilised and in a good position before lifting the heavy object. The seemingly easier tasks of shutting the boot or grabbing your keys require significantly less strength and effort but it's often these activities where we don't think about engaging the supporting structures and the joint is therefore more vulnerable to the fact it's not in an optimal position. Tie this in with the fact we don't often get any pre-warning and it's easy to see how shoulder issues are often niggly and long term in nature because usually, in the initial stages, 99% of the time we're fine. How can you have a shoulder problem yet be able to lift heavy things pain-free? Yet the sharp pain you get when reaching out to get your phone that was just a little bit further out of your reach than you thought is real so there must be something that's not right?

The reality is that something isn't right but it probably isn't where you think it is or where the body is telling you it is. Lots of people will experience pain shooting or referring down the arm or in and around the shoulder blade or the upper back as well as pain within the joint.

People are often drawn to grabbing the upper arm where it hurts or swinging the shoulder around a bit to free it up because they feel it must be stiff if it's hurting and they're starting to get less range of movement in the shoulder. The discomfort and then accompanying restrictions in range of movement are indicators that the shoulder isn't being held in the best place so to then dig around where it hurts or to swing your arm around to try increase the range of movement often irritates the shoulder further. When the shoulder is sore it usually goes into a kind of 'protection mode' where it wants to just do 'safe' movements but this often means that you carry your shoulder a little more rounded. Unfortunately, this further rounding of the shoulder then shortens the anterior muscles further, lengthens the posterior muscles and actually reinforces the issue further by accident. It's another classic snowball scenario whereby a short-term solution actually creates more issues long-term. The short muscles only get shorter, the weak muscles only get weaker, the pain only increases in frequency and intensity and, in the worst cases, people can be left with a shoulder that barely functions. I feel that in the majority of cases that the tide can be turned and you can get the snowball moving in the other direction.

There is often a correlation with shoulder issues whereby the longer pain is experienced, the longer it usually takes to return to pain-free movement so I think it's very important to get to work on shoulder issues as quickly as you can. I'm not suggesting that you panic any time anything hurts but far too often clients will say that they wish they'd come in six months sooner but they didn't think it was an issue because they were fine most of the time and didn't remember doing anything to injure it. That right there is the challenge because the shoulder will often sneak into a suboptimal position without you knowing and you only find out once it starts to hurt. However, if you can understand the main challenges on the shoulders through our day-to-day lives then you have the best chance of ensuring that you can keep your shoulders in the best position they can be through the best stretching and strengthening habits. Let's go through some of these challenges and look at the best ways to counteract them.

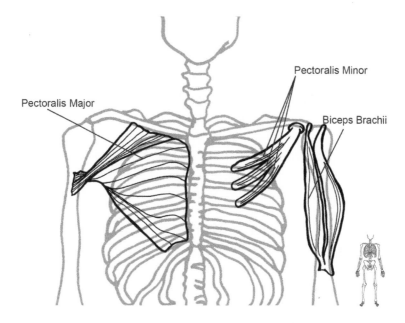

Image 3 – anterior torso and shoulder

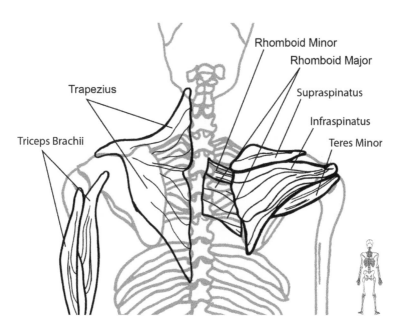

Image 4 – posterior torso and shoulder

Common challenges

Like the upper back and neck, the predominant challenge for shoulders is the anterior versus posterior battle. We don't do a huge amount of activities with our hands behind our backs or with our hands above our heads. We're more likely to find ourselves in positions with our hands out in front of us and reaching down more than up. As per the last chapter this isn't at an all-encompassing list and, again, the list is in no particular order but includes the most common causes (not symptoms) of shoulder pain that I see:

- driving
- using your phone/tablet/smart watch/normal watch
- working at a desk
- sitting on the sofa
- some exercises/sports (especially those where you're predominantly right or left-handed)
- looking after a new born baby/children
- gardening/DIY
- sleeping

As with the last chapter, there will be little tips along the way for each activity and at the end we'll cover the most effective stretches and preventative measures you can take to reduce the stress on your body from these activities. Again, the tips will be ideas to try, not definitive rules, so whenever you try something different make sure you feel confident and safe in doing so.

Driving

Much like the neck and upper back, there is a correlation between the length of time driving and the stress on the shoulders. Additionally, the mechanics involved in actions like changing gear and turning the wheel can frequently highlight underlying issues with the shoulder, be it within the joint itself or with the surrounding muscles. Clients will often explain that they feel like their shoulder 'catches' while they're driving. This catching sensation also includes pain referring down the upper arm, often the outside of the arm, or sharp pains within the joint. This can occur through actions such as changing gear, turning the wheel, raising your arm to say thank you to someone and reaching across to the other seat. Driving is another activity where the arms are out in front of you which naturally causes stress to the posterior chain. This anterior position also reduces the amount of space in the joint capsule, which in turn increases the likelihood of discomfort due to the joint being in a suboptimal position.

Different vehicles can add different stresses to the body. The seating position in a van is different to that of a sports car. If you have an automatic vehicle then you reduce the necessity for gear changes. There are several types of handbrakes and the style you have affects the position of your arm when you apply the handbrake and how much force is required to apply it. The type of driving you do also affects how your body has to function. If you usually find yourself on long motorway drives then you probably won't change gear much. You may also find that you catch yourself slumping down on to the centre console or that you have your arm resting on the arm rest or on the side with the window down. If you are spending more time driving around a busy town, constantly stopping and starting and changing gear, then your body will be working very differently than in the motorway example.

Tips:

- Try to have your arms in as neutral a position on the wheel as possible and as often as possible (there is debate over whether this should be at 10 and 2, 9 and 3 or 8 and 4 so find what is safe and comfortable for you).
- Try to avoid leaning on anything either side of you while driving as this could create more stress on the shoulders.

Using your phone/tablet/smart watch/normal watch

Whichever device you're using the chances are you want to look at it so you won't be using it behind your back too often. Also, it wouldn't be that often that you would need to use any of these items whilst looking up at the sky. So, we find ourselves facing a similar situation with the shoulders to the one with the neck and upper back whereby the anterior and posterior stresses are not equal.

Bringing your wrist towards you to check your watch is not the most strenuous activity going. Even if you have a heavy watch it's not going to replace a gym session any time soon. However, that action repeated numerous times per day, week, month and year will lead to repeated stress on the same side. The same can be said for using your phone. Research numbers fluctuate but at the time of writing it's estimated that the average person checks their phone somewhere around 80–100 times per day. Again, if this task is usually undertaken with the same hand each time then that is a lot more stress to one side of the body. Nowadays, phones and tablets aren't especially heavy but if the weight of the device is usually taken on the same side 100 times per day, day in and day out, one side would be required to work a lot harder than the other. Let's say you often look at your phone or tablet in bed. This example can be switched to either side but let's say you happen to be left-handed, like to lie on your left-hand side in bed (we'll talk more about this in the sleeping section later) watching your tablet which you're holding in your left hand you can see how this action could easily lead to more stress on one shoulder than the other if repeated over time.

Tip:

- Try and swap around which hand you use your devices with and which wrist you wear your watch/smart watch on.

Working at a desk

A lot of the shoulder challenges we face when working at a desk are similar to those of the neck and upper back. The potential for slumping down and rounding is something that we're all too aware of by now. But what about how we use the computer/laptop? If you need to use the number keys frequently and your keyboard has a number keypad on the right, could that mean you'll use your right hand a lot more than your left? If your job requires you to use a mouse frequently then if that is always on the right-hand side will you end up using your right hand more than your left? What about if you need to do writing/notes/drawing as well as using the keyboard? Some people might push their keyboard/laptop further away from them so that they have room to write in front of them but then when you need to use the keyboard you then have to reach further forward to use it. Some people keep the keyboard central and in front of them but then have the paper to the left of the keyboard as the mouse is on the right. If you're right-handed though this would mean leaning across and round in front of you to reach the paper. Even if you don't have a mouse the chances are that if you had to write/draw you would usually use one side more than the other. As always, talking about this isn't designed to get you to never use a computer again but just to get you to think about the patterns that you might be following without even knowing, repeatedly putting the same areas of the body under stress day in and day out.

Tips:

- Get a detachable number keypad so that you don't always use it with one hand more than the other.
- Try swapping the hand that you use the mouse with to make sure that's more balanced.
- Experiment with different mouse styles and find one that suits you best.

Sitting on the sofa

This is another location for the anterior versus posterior challenge to occur. As we've touched on before, sofas generally encourage us to round our shoulders and to slump into a 'comfy' position. If you happen to be using a device while on the sofa this usually exaggerates this rounding of the shoulders further. As with everything have a think about how you use your shoulders while on the sofa. Do you lean on the arm rest and, if so, is it usually the on same side? Do you usually lie on the sofa and, if so, is that usually on the same side? Do you have someone or something that you usually cuddle up to or that you cuddle and, if so, are you usually in the same position each time this happens? Shoulders can quite often be happy once they're in a certain position but it's often when you go to move that they let you know they're not happy and this is a common occurrence when people are sat on the sofa. Seemingly innocuous movements such as reaching to get something or rearranging how you're sat can easily be enough to irritate an already irritated shoulder.

Tips:

- Change how and where you sit on the sofa to ensure you don't get stuck in the same position each time.
- Try and break up how long you're sat on the sofa by lying flat on your back on the floor to give the shoulders time to relax in a neutral position.

Some exercises/sports (especially those where you're predominantly right or left-handed)

As we covered in the neck and upper back section, although sports and exercise are important and good for you they do come with their own postural challenges. If a sport or exercise encourages you to use one hand more than the other (e.g. racket sports, combat sports, throwing actions) then over time this can create or re-emphasise existing imbalances. There are examples within these sports where someone can be more balanced, such as a cricketer who bowls left-handed but bats right-handed or a tennis player who uses a double-handed forehand and backhand but these examples are less common. You could also argue here that bowling and batting are two very different actions as are the forehand and backhand in tennis but they are examples of someone not being completely dominant on one side. However, these are rarities and most of us are more likely to use one arm more than the other in, not just these but most sports. This in turn increases the risk of overuse issues and also of highlighting already existing imbalances within the joint. You may well be unaware that these imbalances are even there but that's what we're trying to get you to think about. Hypothetically, if our shoulders are a bit rounded and are therefore being pulled forward more than they want to be is it then wise to go to the gym or do exercises at home that reinforce this or encourage more rounding of the shoulders/tightening of the already shortened muscles? As per the last chapter I often see the negative effects of doing strengthening exercises that reinforce the anterior chain tightness, such as those which target the chest, biceps and latissimus dorsi (lats). Also, if the shoulder isn't in the optimal position and the rotator cuff muscles are under more stress, then sometimes exercises that aren't anterior dominant can still cause issues. Clients will often say how exercises such as press-ups, planks and side planks irritate their shoulders. Usually, it's not a case of poor technique but it's just the reality that their shoulders aren't in a good enough position to do these exercises and therefore they feel discomfort while doing exercises that should be good for their shoulders.

Tip:

- See if there are any adaptations you can make to any activities/ sports to reduce excess stress on the shoulder (e.g. double hand instead of single hand in tennis, straight arm planks instead of arms bent, single arm overhead press instead of double to ensure one side isn't dominating).

Looking after a new born baby/children

When you're holding a baby or a child then they're usually on your front. Some slings/carriers are designed for the child to be on your back and, as such, the shoulders aren't the primary carrier of the child. If your arms are the primary carrier then they're likely to be in front of you (anterior versus posterior). As the child grows they get heavier and often more wriggly which means your arms have to work even harder to hold the child. When you're carrying the child do you normally carry them on one side more than the other? I haven't found a pattern with clients as to whether it's their dominant or less dominant arm that suffers more from having a child. You might think if you're right-handed that you'd automatically carry a child with your right hand but it's not always the case. In my experience it's not far off a 50/50 split with which arm a right-handed person carries their child with. Some carry them in their right arm as that's their perceived stronger side. Others will predominantly carry them on their left so that they have their right arm free to do other activities. There isn't a right or a wrong option but the best advice would be to alternate as much as possible so that one side doesn't get used a lot more than the other. As we'll see later carrying a child on one side more than the other can also have a massive impact on the lower back and hips.

Aside from getting heavier and more wriggly the baby will eventually start learning to walk. Many people find themselves holding onto their child's hands or having to catch them when they stumble. Both of these actions often have surprise movements attached to them which can irritate a pre-existing shoulder complaint. Some things can't be changed and I'm definitely not advocating that you let your child fall over to save your shoulder but these are just examples of activities that aren't overly strenuous but that can still cause complaint. Even something balanced like pushing a pushchair has been known to irritate shoulders. Whether it's after pushing one up a steep hill, or using a running buggy, or having to grab the pushchair quickly, or the most common issue of getting the pushchair in or out of the car these are all more examples of activities where your arms are out in front of you.

Tip:

- Try and alternate as often as possible which arm you carry your baby/child with (please don't do this if you don't feel confident using your other arm or have an injury/issue that means this might not be a safe choice).

Gardening/DIY

Gardening and DIY projects can result in our bodies being in some odd positions and sometimes for extended periods of time. But those odd positions aren't the only cause of shoulder issues. Something simple such as painting or raking up leaves, while not appearing to be a particularly stressful activity, can just as easily cause irritation. Unless you happen to work as a carpenter or gardener, the chances are that most gardening or DIY activities you undertake aren't tasks that you normally do day-to-day. Factor in that these activities are then usually repetitive in nature and the potential for shoulder irritation becomes clearer. Sometimes the activity might involve lifting or holding something heavy or awkward in size and shape. It may be that it's not something heavy we're lifting but that it's outstretched in front of us (using a hedge trimmer for example). We don't often have our arms above our head during the day so then something like painting a ceiling can be a troublesome activity for many. Again, it's not that the brush or roller is heavy it's just the positions that we have to hold and repeat aren't positions we often take. Similar to most other activities we've already covered, we don't do much gardening or DIY with our arms behind our back. Although, using the painting a ceiling example again, it's not just anterior versus posterior that challenges us here but also the variety of positions in which we can find shoulders. As stated at the start of the chapter, the range of movement our shoulders can reach seems like both a good thing and bad thing at times. It's always amazing what the body can do but sometimes it's not until two days later when you've got a new pain in your shoulder, or when an existing issue has been aggravated, that we realise that maybe we did too much.

Tips:

- Try and take regular breaks to ensure that you're not caught doing a repetitive activity for longer than you realise.
- Try and think about what activity you're doing and whether you need to do it solely with your dominant side. For example, you could sand a door frame left-handed and paint it right-handed or vice versa.
- Make sure you have the correct equipment wherever possible and make sure you're not overextending yourself. Rather than standing on top of the ladder and reaching out as far as you can to save time, try and take that extra minute to go down, readjust the ladder and go back up to reduce the risk of putting excess strain on yourself.

Sleeping

Sleeping is rarely a cause of shoulder issues but it can highlight existing problems. A common scenario is someone struggling with an inflamed rotator cuff tendon, caused by the shoulder being rotated too far forward, that then sleeps on that side at night and gets woken up by the pain. It would be hard to point the finger at sleeping but in this common scenario the sleeping position does reinforce the existing issue. In more chronic situations even lying on the opposite shoulder is just as painful as just the weight of the joint resting is enough of a stress to cause discomfort. On a few occasions, where clients have usually slept with their arms above their heads for example, over a period of months, most have been able to retrain themselves into at least falling asleep in a more neutral position. They will occasionally still wake up with their arms above their heads but a reduction in the frequency of this has definitely had a positive effect on their discomfort levels.

Tip:

- If you think your shoulder position when sleeping could be having a negative impact then see if you can try going to sleep in a different position. I wouldn't expect any instant miracles but it could be that over a period of a few weeks you feel a gradual improvement.

Frozen shoulder

Now, frozen shoulder gets its own section here. It's the elephant in the room that hasn't been mentioned so far. I must stress this is my opinion but I feel the term gets thrown around a lot just to give someone a diagnosis. I feel it's quite generalised and often being given that as your diagnosis can be as useful as someone simply confirming you have shoulder pain. The spectrum of what 'frozen shoulder' can cover is too vast. You can find advice telling you it will go away by itself within one year all the way up to five years. Some people say use heat, others say ice. Anti-inflammatories help. Anti-inflammatories do nothing. You should try to use it to keep it mobile but don't do too much. But what is too much? You could search for 'frozen shoulder exercises' and get bamboozled by all the conflicting information.

I must admit that I have seen a couple of clients over the years who have been in such a bad way that they have turned to having cortisone (anti-inflammatory) injections. They had already been in pain for months and the area was too inflamed for me to make any progress with treatment as it was so we tried the injection to see if it would help. However, there have also been tens of clients who have been told they'd need an injection but, through a combination of treatment, stretching and eventually strengthening, we have been able to avoid that and return them to a full range of movement and function without the need for that intervention. Talking about this always reminds me of when I was training and was called by someone who was desperate. They'd been diagnosed with frozen shoulder, were due surgery in three months and were desperate to try anything to avoid it. I was honest and told her that I was still training but I'd be happy to see if I could help her. When I saw her she told me she'd had the discomfort for a few months, was on painkillers every day and that she was booked on the waiting list for an operation but she'd been told it would be within three months. I asked her how that diagnosis had been formed and she told me it was because of the pain and the fact she couldn't lift her arms past shoulder level. She'd been given the diagnosis a couple of months before and it was getting worse week-by-week. I asked her if anyone had ever actually done any physical treatment or even actually touched her shoulder and she said no. The decision had been made and she was lined up for an operation without having anyone ever physically touch her shoulder. I got her to perform a few basic tests (as that was all I knew at the time) to assess her range of movement. As expected she couldn't get her arms past shoulder level in any range of movement. This didn't look great initially but then I tried an idea I'd just been taught. I got her to close her eyes and I moved her arm and shoulder around to see if I could get any more movement out of it. Immediately I could move her arm just above shoulder level. I then proceeded to do a bit of hands-on treatment on all the muscles in and around the shoulder as I didn't have the knowledge to work on a more targeted or specific area. Half an hour later I retested and got her to see what she could do. She could get her arm just above level by herself which she was chuffed about. I then got her to close her eyes and retested and could get her arm comfortably above level. Long story short I treated her again the following week and by the end of that session she could take her arm comfortably past shoulder level. However, when I got her to close her eyes I could take her arm completely above her head and get complete range of movement in her shoulder. When I got her to open her eyes she couldn't believe that her arm was right above her head.

That quick and dramatic a change is not seen in many clients to be honest but it was a wonderful experience to have while training. It showed for me the importance of doing hands-on treatment as well as the psychology that is involved in pain and injuries. The fear she had around her shoulder was so great because she was consistently being told that because she couldn't do such and such a movement that had meant she had a bad shoulder. But then the fear of having a 'bad shoulder' meant she restricted what she did with it, resulting in it becoming stiffer and more restricted. This is another classic example of the snowball effect in action and almost led to this client having surgery that was realistically unnecessary.

Like we keep saying, shoulders are an extremely complex area of the body but I feel that far too frequently issues get generally diagnosed as 'frozen shoulder' and then accordingly numerous, potentially unnecessary, injections and operations are undertaken when maybe they don't need to be. I've lost count of the amount of clients who have had previous injections or surgery on a 'frozen shoulder' before having treatment and who then mention to me that the other shoulder is starting to play up and ask if I can do anything with it. They often tell me they doubt I'll be able to help as, "This is how the other shoulder started and that ended up needing an operation." But then, when we do get on top of the issue and sort the shoulder out without the need for an operation they then usually say something like, "I probably didn't need the operation on the other shoulder did I?"

I'm not trying to get you to question every diagnosis as I have had a few clients over the years who have needed surgery. However, don't be afraid to question diagnoses and explore other options, as sometimes having an incorrect diagnosis can lead to all sorts of unnecessary stress and discomfort.

General tips

A lot of the tips here interlink with those in the neck and upper back section and have therefore been covered previously. There are a few tips which do stand out though. The first being to take regular breaks when doing activities. Whether it is sport, work, DIY or gardening, taking regular breaks and not doing activities relentlessly gives you a chance to rest and reset before going again. Tied in with this is the challenge of trying not to use your dominant hand all the time. Just the simple thought, "Do I need to be doing this with this hand?" can be enough to make a massive difference to the balance and efficiency of your body over time.

Finally, don't let a label or diagnosis define how you use your shoulders. So often it's the case that after receiving a diagnosis clients will be scared to use their shoulders and will overprotect them. They will often refer to it as their 'bad shoulder' therefore giving it a label. This in turn can lead to even further reduction of the range of movement and potentially even more discomfort. You can't just override your brain and pretend something is fine if it's not but similarly it's important not to stress yourself into more pain. Along the same lines I would always advise injections and surgery as a last resort. Try and explore all options before committing to something like that. I fear that thousands of avoidable injections and operations take place every year. If there is inflammation in and around the shoulder then why is that the case? Does hitting the symptom with an intense burst of anti-inflammatory sort out the problem of why it was inflamed in the first place? If your shoulder is sitting too far forward in the joint and reducing the space in the joint capsule because of anterior muscles that are too strong and posterior muscles that are too weak does shaving some of your bone away to make more space in the joint get to the root of the problem?

If you've tried all possible avenues and are left with no other choice, then of course injections and surgery have their place but it might not always be what's needed.

What not to do

It makes sense to talk about the anterior versus posterior challenge first as it has been a common theme throughout. If the muscles of the anterior chain are too strong and short, as is the case for most people, then strengthening these further will only exacerbate the imbalance. Therefore, chest and bicep strengthening specifically can often have a negative impact on shoulder alignment and stability.

Tied in with this stretching the upper back muscles (essentially rounding your shoulders even more) should generally be avoided as we don't want to encourage further lengthening of potentially already weak and overstretched muscles.

If you are experiencing shoulder discomfort then I think it's really important not to try and 'free up' the shoulder by swinging it around or trying to challenge the range of movement yourself. If you have been given specific advice to try and challenge the shoulder in a specific direction then this is different but generally if the joint or surrounding structures are irritated then they won't react positively to being stretched, pulled and swung into positions that they don't want to go. Also, unless you know specifically what needs to be worked on after seeking advice, don't poke around or rub the shoulder. Quite often we're drawn to poking or rubbing the bit that's sore and, as is often the case, that's usually the area that is likely to be inflamed, so if you go digging around you can accidentally create further stress and inflammation yourself. I often see clients who have been experiencing pain down the outside of their upper arm. This can often be caused by rotator cuff inflammation but the pain itself is felt as referred pain down the arm. Many clients have come in with bruises on their upper arm from where they have been poking and prodding where the pain has been when actually the issue is elsewhere. So, as always, if in doubt leave it alone.

What to do

This can be slightly trickier with shoulders as it depends how the shoulder is feeling in the first place. The initial advice is given to be on the assumption that the shoulder is fine and symptom free. If this is the case then posterior chain strengthening is always advised. Strengthening the muscles of the upper back helps to retract the shoulders and keep the joint in a more neutral position. Similarly, increasing the strength in the rotator cuff muscles helps massively with keeping the shoulders back and stabilised. In terms of combatting the anterior shortening, chest stretching is always a winner as this helps to open up the front of the joint and reduce the stresses and strains of pulling the shoulder forward.

However, the advice changes slightly if you have existing discomfort with your shoulder and depends on the severity of this discomfort. For example, if you have chronic shoulder pain due to rotator cuff tendonitis then, initially, rotator cuff strengthening should be avoided. As strengthening is a form of stress on an area, if that area is already under a lot of stress then it's ill-advised to add further stress. Similarly, although chest stretching is massively important to helping encourage the shoulders to retract, certain chest stretches can cause discomfort in the joint if the shoulder is already inflamed. It might be an obvious point but if you are stretching your chest out then you want to feel the stretch in the chest muscles. If you are stretching your chest and all you can feel is pain referring down your upper arm then it's not the right stretch to be doing right now. It would need to be adapted to make sure that you're not accidentally adding more stress to the area. As always, if you're not sure then seek advice as it's always a shame when you think you're doing something to help yourself and in fact it turns out you were actually making things worse by accident.

Other factors

It's worth a mention, as per the last chapter, that sometimes there are issues that treatment, stretching and strengthening can't fully solve. The most common structural issues in this category are bone spurs and joint calcification. Here, injections and/or surgery can be necessary if a full range of movement and pain-free movement can't be achieved. However, in over a decade I can count the number of clients on one hand where this has been the case so it doesn't come up that frequently. Likewise, a shoulder dislocation is another example where further interventions would be required but this situation is usually quite self-explanatory as you can often see, let alone feel, that this injury has occurred.

CHAPTER 5

Elbows, Forearms and Wrists

Much like with the shoulder, feeling pain in and around the elbow and wrist can be concerning. Whether it's one or the other or both, it's not a nice feeling. Often people experience nerve discomfort and sometimes numbness in the fingers. None of these experiences are pleasant but most are often avoidable. We'll cover each of these in more depth later on but the most common complaints associated with this area are often diagnosed as Carpal Tunnel Syndrome, tennis elbow and golfer's elbow. These diagnoses, as well as most others, are usually arrived at after a sustained period of discomfort. It's rare but not unheard of for pain around the elbows, forearms and wrists to be acute in nature. However, more often than not, it's the case that through a combination of repetitive activities and muscular imbalance an area will be consistently put under stress until it reaches a tipping point and we experience pain. These repetitive activities may involve actions such as gripping, rotating and typing among others but they don't always have to be especially strenuous. Actions such as moving a mouse around at your desk or typing on a keyboard or gripping a paintbrush wouldn't be classed as extreme sports by most but if done continuously and compounded over time, these activities can be major contributors to discomfort and pain.

So far, the anterior versus posterior challenge has featured heavily throughout this book and it's back again here. When we look at the elbows and wrists we are often looking at the relationship between the flexor muscles and extensor muscles of the forearm. During day-to-day life, as well as for many activities that we undertake using our hands, we generally find our wrists and elbows will spend more time in flexion than extension. Although there are a number of situations where the muscle groups will be working isometrically (equally against each other) the predominant position is flexion. Let's look at using a computer mouse or typing as an example. Although the wrist itself isn't being flexed much we still flex our fingers to hold, move or click the mouse or while tapping the keys when typing. We'd also likely have our elbow slightly bent when doing these activities which would again involve shortening of the flexor muscles and lengthening of the extensor muscles. We'll go through the most common challenges shortly, how they can lead to discomfort and how best to avoid them with some useful tips.

I don't want to sound like I'm going along the 'challenge every diagnosis' route again but I suppose I'm saying you don't have to always accept the diagnosis and resulting interventions that are suggested as set in stone. I've lost count of the number of clients, either new or existing, who just drop into the conversation something like,

Did I tell you I'm being booked in for an operation for my Carpal Tunnel? I've been told there's nothing that can be done for it apart from the surgery. There's no point in you looking at it is there?

I don't know why but for some reason the wrists and elbows seem to be an area of the body that people think can't be treated, or that it's pointless being looked at. Maybe it's because so many get told that nothing else will work apart from an operation or injection. I don't know what it is but my answer is always the same – "Let's have a look and see what we can find."

There are significant similarities here to the 'frozen shoulder' dilemma. I've seen so many clients who have the scar on one wrist from a Carpal Tunnel operation and are either booked in or lined up for the same operation on the other wrist. However, through a combination of treatment on the wrist flexor muscles, as well as making a few tweaks to some of the main activities that challenge their wrist, the vast majority have been able to avoid the second operation. Of course, that in turn leads to the inevitably awkward question of, "If we got this one sorted out do you think I actually needed the operation on the other one in the first place?" There's never a simple answer to that question as the circumstances could well have been different and people do need surgery sometimes. However, if the symptoms were the same on both sides and one side had an operation and one side had treatment and stretching with the end result being the same then there could be an argument as to whether the original operation was actually necessary. My hope would be that if you are reading this as someone who has been told there's nothing that can be done and are awaiting surgery, you explore some hands-on therapy to see if you can get an improvement and avoid a potentially unnecessary operation. All operations carry risk, however quick and simple they may be, so in my opinion I would always consider them as a last resort. I'm also not saying that Carpal Tunnel Syndrome isn't a real issue but I would say I disagree with how quickly and often surgery is recommended as the solution. Let's look at the primary muscles involved with the most common elbow, forearm and wrist issues.

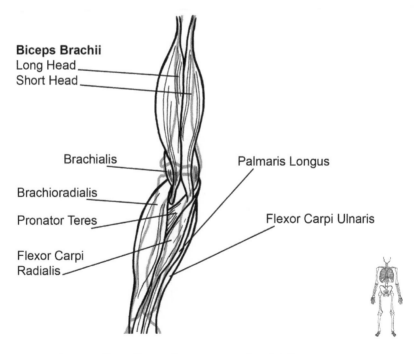

Image 5 – elbow, forearm and wrist flexors

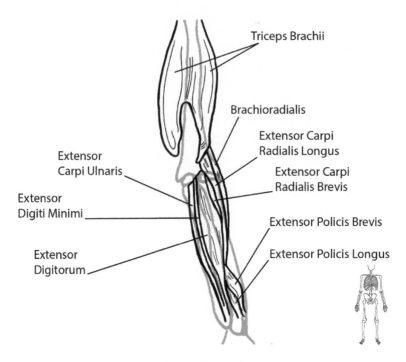

Triceps Brachii

Brachioradialis

Extensor Carpi
Radialis Longus

Extensor Carpi
Radialis Brevis

Extensor
Carpi Ulnaris

Extensor
Digiti Minimi

Extensor Policis Brevis

Extensor Policis Longus

Extensor
Digitorum

Image 6 – elbow, forearm and wrist extensors

Common challenges

As in the last chapter, this isn't at an all-encompassing list and, again, the list is in no particular order but these are the most common causes (not symptoms) of elbow, forearm and wrist pain that I see:

- driving
- cycling
- using your phone/tablet
- working at a desk
- some exercises/sports (especially those where you're predominantly right or left-handed)
- looking after a new born baby/children
- gardening/DIY
- physical jobs
- playing musical instruments
- sleeping

Driving

I mentioned earlier that an activity doesn't have to be especially strenuous to cause stress and driving is a classic example of this. The range of movement we take our elbows, wrists and forearms through while driving aren't especially drastic. However, we are required to have constant tension in these muscle groups to ensure we have a strong enough grip on the steering wheel to maintain control of the vehicle. Like most activities that involve gripping, the flexor and extensor muscles have to work in synchronisation. However, this synchronisation often involves the flexors being a touch shorter and tighter and the extensors a touch longer and overstretched. To grip we have to close our fists slightly which is where the flexors have the potential to tighten up as this requires them to shorten. If you have a manual vehicle then you can also add in the action of changing gear which again requires gripping and flexing. Most clients don't experience any sharp pains from driving as the issues tend to be chronic in nature. A few gear changes and a five-minute drive aren't going to change the world but the same actions, repeated over months, years or even decades, can eventually lead to stress and irritation. It would be rare to see a specific injury in this circumstance or a specific incident that caused instant pain so most people will overlook driving as a significant contributing factor to their discomfort.

Tip:

- Try to break up long drives to reduce the relentlessness of gripping the steering wheel.

Cycling

Cycling is also often overlooked as a cause of elbow, forearm and wrist discomfort. Cycling is usually a cause of more acute discomfort but this doesn't mean that it shouldn't also be considered a contributing factor to chronic discomfort. I've had many a conversation with a client starting with, "My forearms feel really tired and sore and I've got no idea why." Yet a couple of minutes later we discover they've been on a mammoth ride on their road bike the previous weekend or had randomly fancied a bit of downhill mountain biking a few days ago. Similar to numerous other examples covered in this book, the challenge here is that there is rarely discomfort while doing the action itself. Be it gripping the handlebars, squeezing the brakes or changing gear – all these actions require functional and controlled movements. If you're out for a few hours on a 60-mile ride on your road bike this will inevitably tire the muscles. But the specific muscles used and fatigue experienced will be slightly different to someone who has done some downhill mountain biking where they may well be gripping harder, changing gear less and squeezing the brake more and probably for longer periods of time. So, although both activities come under the umbrella of cycling the stresses and strains they put on the body will be slightly different. However, both activities require the flexors to be working slightly shorter and the extensors slightly overstretched. Looking at the elbow position, in both activities, the elbows are likely to spend more time in a flexed position (arms bent) more so than extended (straight arms). This is even more likely with downhill biking as it's often argued that the flexed arm position helps with shock absorption and is better at reducing tension and fatigue in the muscles. This is a classic example of adapting to the scenario but also shows how flexion isn't always a bad thing and can help to reduce stress elsewhere in the body.

Tip:

- Try to break up long rides with regular breaks.

Using your phone/tablet

For many of us this an area where prolonged and repetitive usage can occur. It's easy to find yourself flicking through your phone for what seems like five minutes to then look up and find half an hour has gone by. However you flick through your phone the chances are that you use one hand more than the other. The other likelihood is that your elbows and wrists will be flexed more often than extended. Not many of us use our devices with our arms outstretched in front of us. Nor do we use the devices with our thumbs and fingers extended and spread out. It's quite hard to get creative enough to think of different ways to use your phone or tablet so the common sense approach of trying not to use any device for too long comes back in to play again here.

Tips:

- Try not to be on your device for extended periods of time.
- Try and swap around which hand you use your devices with to make sure you're sharing the load.

Working at a desk

It's hard not to sound like a broken record in this chapter but here we go again. When we are sat at a desk and using a computer it's likely that we'll have our arms slightly bent rather than locked out straight. We mentioned this earlier but, like in many other activities, the mechanics of typing mean that we spend more time with the flexors shortened and the extensors lengthened. This results in neither muscle group functioning at their optimal length and usually for prolonged periods of time. An extra factor to consider with typing is the pressure that is put through your elbows and forearms from resting them on the desk. Initially this may seem pretty trivial as it's hardly like there's a huge amount of body weight going through your bones in that position. However, even light pressure compounded over time can lead to discomfort. If you're someone who leans on an arm rest of the chair or slumps down on one elbow on your desk then the forces put through the joint will be even higher. As always, I'm not trying to pick holes in everything or make every activity sound dangerous, I'm just trying to get you to think about how you use your body day in and day out and how seemingly minor stresses can add up when compounded over time.

Tips:

- Try to take regular breaks from sitting in the same position at the desk.
- If you're resting your elbows/forearms on a firm surface you could change this to something a little softer.
- Try not to slump/lean down on one arm rest. If you are someone that does this then you could try changing to a chair without armrests to remove the temptation.

Some exercises/sports (especially those where you're predominantly right or left-handed)

It seems sensible to start here with activities that involve gripping. After all, the two most 'famous' elbow issues are named after sports but we'll cover golfer's and tennis elbow a bit later on. We could write a whole chapter just breaking down the effects of every sport on the elbow, forearms and wrists so I'm just going to pick a few examples. Anything that involves using a bat, club, racquet or stick is going to involve a lot of gripping and possibly on one side more than the other. Any activity that requires a throwing or bowling action will require a controlled grip and usually on one side more than the other. Many sports may require more equal gripping such as cycling and rowing. Some activities require gripping for extended periods of time such as rock climbing or bouldering. Moving away from gripping, swimming deserves a mention as although no gripping is involved the wrists are in a flexed position to allow efficient movement through the water. Diving is a sport where the wrists are stressed massively but in a very different way due to the impact of hitting the water.

When it comes to exercise a lot of weight training activities involve gripping of the relevant equipment (such as a dumbbell, barbell, tyre, rope, sandbag and kettlebell). As per the running theme of this chapter these gripping activities can often lead to shorter, tighter flexors and longer, overstretched extensors. Linked into this is the fact that many clients mention that they suffer discomfort when they do press-ups or burpees. Interestingly, these are a couple of the few activities that involve the wrist being in an extended rather than flexed position. For many, this position irritates the wrist as it's a combination of it being a weight-bearing action in a position in which we don't find ourselves that often.

Tips:

- Don't lift heavier weights than you can manage.
- Try not to do any activity to excess.
- Try to use both hands rather than just one side or, if you can, alternate which hand is your dominant – although this is not always that practical in reality.

Looking after a new born baby/children

When carrying a baby or child we tend not to have our arms and wrists locked out straight. Not only would that look strange but it wouldn't be especially safe. Whether you're cradling, feeding or carrying a child your elbow and wrist will usually be flexed to ensure you've got them in the most safe and secure position. This is yet another action that reinforces the anterior shortening and posterior lengthening scenario that we face in so many other activities. The child's comfort and safety are of paramount importance of course so I don't want you experimenting with a strange carrying technique that puts anyone at risk. However, if you feel comfortable to do so, I do recommend regularly swapping which arm you carry the child with. If you were bottle feeding, for example, you could try to alternate which hand you feed them with so that you don't always repeat the same pattern. Linking this back to the interconnectivity of the body, if you always held them in your left arm while feeding them with your right hand then you're also always going to be looking the same way down at them, so you can see how this could also have an impact on neck and shoulder imbalance. Babies only get heavier and wrigglier as time goes by so the earlier you can get into a good habit of alternating and feeling confident with carrying them on either side the better.

Tips:

- Using a sling/carrier instead of carrying the child in your arms will take the stress off the forearms.
- As long as you feel confident try to alternate which arm you hold your child with, be that while feeding or just carrying them around.

Gardening/DIY

Similar to the exercise and sports section above there are countless different activities that could be mentioned here. I would say painting is the biggest danger sport in the DIY section here. The repetitive nature and prolonged gripping are the main reasons for this. Sanding is probably a close second as the two often come hand-in-hand. Activities such as hammering and sawing also feature prominently for the same reasons of repetitive and prolonged use. Moving on to gardening and digging is probably the main cause of discomfort. Whether using a spade, shovel or small trowel, the act of digging requires controlled gripping and repetitive movements. Here you can also get the unexpected vibrations and stress from hitting a rock or ground that is harder than expected. For others mowing the lawn causes significant discomfort due to the pushing, pulling and gripping required to direct and run the mower. Using a hedge trimmer or strimmer can be a challenge in terms of prolonged usage, sometimes having to reach out at awkward angles and having to control small, accurate movements while carrying a potentially heavy machine. Many projects incorporate a combination of these actions and stresses. Activities such as laying new decking in the garden or putting up a new fence involve repetitive actions such as digging, sawing, hammering and drilling. So it's easy to see why I often get calls on a Monday from clients who feel tired and broken after their weekend DIY project! In all seriousness, most of these activities do follow the same process of shortening the wrist and elbow flexors. Not many of these activities lead you to have your wrist extended so the potential for repetitive overuse is clear but, as per usual, it's often one of these activities that is a tipping point rather than the sole cause of pain.

Tips:

- Try to alternate which hand you are using as long as it feels safe.
- Try not to do any activity for extended periods of time.

Physical jobs

Many of the physical challenges that we mentioned in the gardening/ DIY section are relevant here. All jobs have some sort of physical element to them but in this section I'm thinking back to clients I've seen over the years from all sorts of work backgrounds that have had specific and significant issues with their elbows, forearms and wrists. The common link, as expected, is that these jobs often include repetitive actions being undertaken using one hand more than the other. We've already touched on it but let's start with gardeners. You tend to have a dominant hand/side for activities like digging or raking. Mowing the lawn should be fairly equal but if the lawn mower requires you to grip one lever to keep the mower going then that extra stress could add up over time. The same can be said for hedge trimming in terms needing to grip a lever to function the machine itself. Most people will also feel more comfortable holding it a certain way with one hand being more dominant over the other. Moving on to carpenters and roofers, most will feel more comfortable using a saw or hammer with one hand over the other. I've seen many bricklayers with elbow issues due to the repetitive nature of the activity, along with the fact that as the bricks themselves can be an awkward size the gripping of them can be uncomfortable. Most bricklayers will have a rhythm and prefer working a certain way but this same activity compounded over time does put more stress on one side more than the other. Plasterers will usually have a preferred hand to work with. Yet again, this is a relentlessly repetitive action. I have met a couple of plasterers who have taught themselves how to do it with their less dominant arm but this is only because they have been in so much pain with their dominant arm that they've had to in order to be able to continue working. I've also had a few chefs over the years with elbow pain. Be it from chopping or using tongs, these are both repetitive actions which repeated relentlessly over days, weeks and months have potential to cause discomfort. As always, one action by itself isn't a massive issue but it's the repetition compounded over time that is the bigger factor. Add this to other factors we've discussed and the compounding effects of the snowball grow and grow.

Tip:
- Can you **safely** do some of your job requirements with your less dominant hand? For example, if you are a chef please don't start trying to chop with your less dominant hand if you don't feel confident!

Playing musical instruments

Initially, this might sound an odd one because musical instruments aren't often associated with relentless stress but if you dig a little deeper you can see how overuse injuries can occur. If we start with probably the most strenuous activity, drumming, you can imagine how the relentless gripping of the sticks and beating the drums will create tension and tightness over time. I don't actually play any instruments myself so I'm suggesting drumming as the most strenuous based on what I've seen with clients. You may well have other ideas depending on what instrument you play! If you look at the mechanics of playing most instruments there's usually an element of gripping, moving your fingers or often both. Although there may not be many individually physically strenuous movements involved, the relentless, intricate repetition can create fatigue and shortening of the flexor muscles. If you think about the actions involved in playing the piano for example, the stresses are similar to those of typing on a computer keyboard. Playing a guitar also requires relentless gripping and movement. As always, the list can go on and on and we're not going to go through every instrument but the idea here again is that some activities are more stressful on our bodies than we give them credit for.

Tip:

- Take regular breaks to reduce the risks of overuse. Especially when you're learning something new as it's easy to get caught up practicing and not notice how long you've been doing the same activity for so make sure you give yourself regular breaks.

Sleeping

Sleeping makes an appearance once again here but in a similar context to previous chapters. If sleeping is to be considered a factor it's usually highlighting something that's already there as opposed to being the sole cause of the issue. It's not set in stone with everybody but generally we tend to sleep with our wrists slightly flexed and elbows slightly bent. As always, we do move around at night and everybody sleeps slightly differently so this is a generalisation. If you already had short flexor muscles due to activities throughout the day then keeping your wrists flexed when at rest could possibly reinforce this shortening. As with previous body parts and sleeping the tricky part is that we're asleep so we don't know exactly what we're doing or how to change it. For people suffering with extreme discomfort splints or braces are sometimes recommended as they force the wrist to remain in a neutral position. Although some clients have found the splint/brace to be a nuisance that affects their ability to get to sleep, on the whole I've seen that it has helped and complimented the majority of clients in assisting with some pain relief.

Tip:

- If you are finding that sleeping is making the pain worse or you're being woken up at night then splints, braces and supports could be worth a try.

Carpal tunnel syndrome

Carpal Tunnel Syndrome is caused by compression of the median nerve in your forearm. This can lead to numbness, pain and weakness and is generally an unpleasant issue to have to deal with. Although on some occasions it can be caused due to an injury to the wrist, the discomfort usually occurs due to repetitive actions, many of which we have covered in this chapter. Some people find the discomfort worse at night while others find it during the day when they are using their hands. Diagnostic imaging and nerve conduction tests are often used to confirm that the nerve is irritated. The recommended advice is often dependent upon how chronic the issue is. It can start with simple rest, wearing a splint at night and trying to adapt how you work, all the way through to painkillers, steroid injections and even surgery. As always, surgery does have its place in extreme circumstances but this should always been seen as a last resort.

Over the years I have helped numerous clients avoid surgery through a combination of treatment, stretches and sometimes use of splints/braces. As mentioned earlier in the chapter a few of those I've helped had already had surgery on one wrist and just assumed that they'd need surgery on the other side when that started hurting as well. Similar to those who've had frozen shoulder surgery once they get improvements and avoid surgery on their wrist they will then often ask my opinion on whether they should have had the surgery on the original wrist. Because there are numerous factors at work it's not as simple as saying, "This side got better with treatment so the other side would have as well." The most significant factor being that most of us use one hand more than the other every day so the wear and tear and fatigue is rarely equal. However, when you do see someone improve with one wrist it does make you wonder, so I suppose I'm back to the aforementioned point of making sure you explore all options before injections and surgery. Is your setup at work the best it could be? Do you have enough breaks throughout the day? Are there any changes that could be made in your day-to-day life that could reduce the stress on your hands and wrists? Have you tried everything you can to make sure the nerve is under less stress or are you jumping into an injection or surgery because it's a quick fix?

Tennis elbow and golfer's elbow

Although these are two different issues I've put them together here for convenience as there are a number of similarities. Tennis elbow affects the outside of the elbow (lateral epicondylitis) and golfer's elbow affects the inside of the elbow (medial epicondylitis). Both are often caused by overuse/repetitive movements. Interestingly, over the years, I wouldn't say that golf or tennis are anywhere near the most common causes of these issues. Only a handful of clients I've seen with tennis or golfer's elbow have actually played tennis or golf. The reason for telling you this is that you may have thought, "I didn't think it could be that because I don't play tennis/golf." Again, many of the most common causes of these issues have been covered already in this chapter. Alongside treatment tennis elbow straps can be useful at reducing discomfort. Where the discomfort usually arises from tight muscles pulling against the attachments and causing the inflammation (epicondylitis), the straps can sometimes assist in reducing the 'pulling' effect from the muscles and therefore reducing the stress on the attachments.

Another approach that, in my opinion, often gets used a little too quickly is a cortisone (steroid) injection. Although the principle of the injection makes sense, to attempt to reduce the inflammation, if nothing else changes then the cause of the issue is likely to still remain and, even if the injection is successful at reducing pain levels, the issue has every chance of returning again. Don't get me wrong, these injections do have their place and I have seen a couple of clients where the inflammation/issue was so chronic (i.e. they'd been in pain for many, many months before doing anything about it) that I recommended that they give the injection a try. However, I do feel this should be used as a last resort not the first step and through a combination of treatment, temporary adaptations (e.g. using your phone a bit less for a while or wearing a support strap) and permanent adaptations (e.g. changing your workplace setup with a different chair/desk/keyboard) the necessary improvements can be made to reduce the stress on the attachments and thus reduce the inflammation and pain. Where the pain usually sneaks in over a period of weeks or months, as opposed to just coming on one day, it can be easy to just hope it goes away by itself so I'd always recommend getting advice or treatment for it sooner rather than later.

General tips

In summary, there are a couple of key points to think about with the elbows, forearms and wrists. Firstly, whether it be work, gardening, DIY or sports are you set up as efficiently as possible or are there any changes that could be made, big or small, that could benefit you in making sure there's no unnecessary stress going through your elbows, forearms and wrists?

Secondly, always try and take regular breaks to reduce overuse issues. Even if that means setting an alarm so you don't forget so be it. You might be having a nice time pottering in the garden and then, before you know it, you've been painting or digging for two hours straight. This leads nicely into the last point of remembering that you have two hands so, if you can and if it's safe to do so, try using your less dominant hand as often as you can. Remember, safety is important here so you may find you need to practice and you may well find with some activities it just won't be practical to use the less dominant hand. But if you can spread the load and use your body in the most balanced way you can then you will definitely feel better for doing so.

What not to do

If it hurts leave it alone. If you have pain on the inside or outside of your elbow, or if you're really unlucky both, then the pain is there due to inflammation. So poking, prodding and rubbing it is only likely to cause more discomfort. If your fingers feel numb then wiggling them more to 'wake them up' will often lead to more tightness in the muscles that are causing the issue. If your wrist feels stiff or sore the chances are that rotating it around or flexing it back and forth is probably using the very same muscles that are causing you the discomfort in the first place.

What to do

Where the main muscles of the forearm run longitudinally (from elbow to wrist) then gripping, squeezing and twisting the muscles side-to-side can be a very effective way of separating the fibres and relieving tension. Also, by twisting the skin in two different directions simultaneously you can maximise the effect of the technique. As it's often the flexor muscles that are tight stretching these can often be useful. However, if you have pain at the wrist then this could actually cause more discomfort so, as always, if in doubt seek professional advice. In the same mould extensor strengthening can be beneficial in some scenarios but, if you were experiencing tennis elbow symptoms for example, it wouldn't be advised so again seek professional advice before doing that.

If you are experiencing pain from inflammation then simply applying an ice pack to the area can help to reduce discomfort but remember that this is only helping ease the symptoms and not addressing the overall cause. The same can be said for splints, braces, straps and kinesiology tape. These all have a suitable time and place for use but the key factor is always to try and determine the cause of the discomfort and work towards making changes there rather than just continually firefighting the symptoms.

Other factors

As per previous chapters there will always be some factors that are more difficult to control. With wrists and elbows especially, hypermobility in the joints can cause stress to the surrounding muscles, ligaments and tendons so adequate strengthening to improve the joint stability is hugely important here. Also, all the hands-on treatment in the world isn't going to fix a stress fracture or broken bone so if there's any possibility of either of these being a factor then these should be explored thoroughly through relevant imaging scans.

CHAPTER 6

Hips and Lower Back

We put our hips and lower back through a lot of stress and many structures have to work together to allow us to have that magical balance of movement while maintaining stability. The hips and the spine are capable of an extraordinary range of movement but to do this they require the stability of a multitude of muscles, ligaments and tendons. It's amazing that we don't over-flex, over-extend or over-rotate more often when you think about the positions that we get ourselves into sometimes. Just think about what has to happen for you to simply squat down and pick up a pen that you've dropped, for example. Unfortunately, it's often simple movements such as those that can be the tipping point for back and hip issues to occur. We're often unaware that we're out of balance side-to-side, anterior to posterior or, more than likely, a combination of the two until something goes wrong. On rare occasions I've seen clients that have lifted something far too heavy, or far heavier than they expected and it's got them into trouble. However, far more frequently, it's seemingly innocuous activities like putting the lead on the dog, picking up a plastic bag or reaching down to pick up your phone that ends up leading to back spasms. The common theme in near enough every back issue of this type is the fact the spine is flexed forwards and the posterior muscles are overstretched (i.e. you're leaning forward rather than backward). The brain decides at that point that the spine can't be overstretched any further and the muscles spasm and you 'lock up' as a form of self-preservation. After all, the brain doesn't want to risk any potential damage to the spinal cord. However, what most people do next can often do more harm than good. If the brain has decided that protection is the best play at this point and has intentionally stiffened you up to reduce the risk of damage, then why does it feel so good to stretch your back at this point? This is yet another example of 'if it hurts don't stretch it' however much it might feel like the right thing to do. Most people will try and touch their toes, or at least lean forward and possibly try and rotate their hips to 'free up' the back. It's almost a reflex reaction for most people to the stiffening up but it's not what the body needs. If you imagine that the area is in a bit of a panic/self-protection mode then you can see how adding more stress to it by trying to stretch it out further, often recreating the very movement that just caused you the pain in the first place, isn't the best approach. If you touched something hot and it burned your finger and then you went back and touched it again or even held your finger on the hot surface for even longer, you wouldn't expect a better outcome. For me, this is one of the biggest changes that people have to make and something that I often get a lot of resistance with.

The classic question, "If it's the wrong thing to do then why does it feel so nice?" often comes out again here. It's been the common theme throughout but stretching something that is already overstretched is going to make things worse. You feel pain because the nerves are under stress. If you stretch it further you will feel more nerve pain but that isn't doing you any good. As always, it's the muscles that are keeping quiet that you need to be thinking about here. The key to happy hips and backs is balance. Balance between left and right and balance between front and back. Sounds easy. But in reality how many activities do we do, day-to-day or through exercise/sports, where our hips and lower backs are in equal balance? Bonus points if you thought of standing up straight or doing a plank. Anyone who has ever had a treatment with me will testify that I rave about both of those activities all the time for the very reason that everything is working in equilibrium – left working equally against right, front working equally against back. However, in the vast majority of actions and activities we undertake throughout any given day our bodies will not be equal.

If we think about the key muscular players here they are all trying to work to keep you neutral and balanced. If something shortens up one side then there has to be a reaction from the other side. The best way in which I try and get people to visualise this is to get them to think about the pelvis. In an ideal world all the muscles around the pelvis are pulling equally to maintain a neutral position (like when standing up straight or doing a plank). The dominant muscles I see frequently affecting the tilt of the pelvis are the hamstrings on the back and the hip flexors on the front. I say dominant muscles here because other muscles are definitely involved, principally the gluteal muscles (glutes) which are the main powerhouse for maintaining stability. Hopefully, the following analogy will help you to see where I'm coming from.

This may seem strange but let's imagine the pelvis as a square see-saw. Label one corner of the see-saw as front right, one as front left, one as back right and one as back left. Now imagine four equally-sized piles of four bricks on each of the four corners. Hopefully, you can visualise that the see-saw would be balanced as the forces are equal in each corner. Let's mess around with the bricks and see what happens. If we took all the bricks from the back left and added them to the front left and then did the same with the back right and added them to the front right the see-saw would tilt forward with an anterior tilt. In muscular terms this is the equivalent of the hip flexors being too short and tight and the hamstrings being too overstretched and weak. If we flip this around and now put all the bricks equally to the back left and the back right then the see-saw would tilt backward with a posterior tilt. Here the hamstrings would be too short and tight and dominating against the over stretched hip flexor muscles. You may or may not have heard of the terms anterior and posterior tilt but I've seen so many clients that have been told they have one or the other. The reality I've seen over the years is that both are relatively rare. If one were more common than the other then I'd say I've seen more posterior tilts but the reality is to have true anterior or posterior tilt means that you would have to be completely equal between left and right and that is definitely a rarity. I would very seldom meet someone with very tight and equally tight hip flexors and very overstretched and equally overstretched hamstrings (anterior tilt) or vice versa (posterior tilt). Let's go back to the see-saw analogy.

Imagine we're back at the start with four bricks on each of the four corners. What would happen if you just took all the bricks from the front left and added them to the front right while leaving the bricks at the back alone? The see-saw would tilt forward and to the right a bit so how would you balance that up at the back to make the see-saw neutral again? You'd have to take all the bricks from the back right and add them to the bricks on the back left. Now, in this example, you've got all the weight on the front right balancing off against all the weight on the back left but yet the see-saw is still in balance. Muscularly this isn't possible of course because that would mean you don't have any left hip flexor or right hamstring muscles so let's tweak your see-saw a little bit to make it more accurate. I want you to take two of the bricks from the front left and put them on the front right so you're left with six on the front right and two on the front left. Now, at the back I want you to take two of the bricks from the back right and move them to the back left so that you're left with six on the back left and two on the back right. What do you think you'd be left with? Although you'd still be in balance there'd be more pressure on the front right and back left. This is the equivalent of the right hip flexor and left hamstring being tighter than their opposites but technically you'd still be balanced at this point. However, the long-term effect of this extra pressure on different points of the see-saw/pelvis could eventually start to take its toll and you might expect the front right of the see-saw to start to drop eventually and likewise the back left due to the extra pressure. But what if you added even more stress to the situation? How about if I told you that you had an extra pile of bricks next to the see-saw and every week you had to add one new brick to the front right pile and one new brick to back left pile? These areas would still be counterbalancing each other but the cumulative stress on the see-saw would be increasing week-by-week. You'd start to see the see-saw dropping even more towards the front right and towards the back left.

Now we're being more realistic about what most of us are like. To be clear, it's just as common to be the opposite way round (short left hip flexors and short right hamstrings) but most people have one side at the front that's tighter (either the right or left hip flexors) and then usually the opposite side on the back that's tighter (either the left or right hamstrings) to counterbalance. This continual counterbalance stress eventually leads to the pelvis being rotated/twisted (i.e. not neutral and balanced) but not equally forward or backward and not equally one side over the other. It's this rotation and lack of balance that often puts stress on one hip more than the other or one side of the lower back over the other.

Clients will often say that their back pain is presenting as 'right in the middle' but when you explore the muscles either side of the spine you often find that one side is short and tight and one side is overstretched and that it's the overstretched side that, when worked on, recreates the pain they've been feeling. One way to bring this to life is to imagine yourself standing up but leaning on your left leg/hip. Most people will lean on one hip more than the other while standing anyway and most people aren't even consciously aware that they do it. By putting more weight on the left leg the left hamstrings will tighten up to help stabilise you. But then, to counterbalance, you'll find yourself bending the right knee slightly and therefore shortening up the right hip flexors to try and get the pelvis back to as neutral a place as possible. However, this is still a rotated pelvis. If you were more likely to lean on your right hip then the opposite muscles would shorten up and you'd end up with tighter right hamstrings and left hip flexors.

HUGE TIP – *I know the tips are usually saved for later but this is too important to wait! When you're stood up if you try tensing your glutes/ buttocks equally for a couple of seconds you'll find that helps to reset you and balance up your pelvis. That's an important thing to work on especially if you are one of life's leaners. It won't change overnight but the stronger you get and more used to being neutral you become, the less stress you put on your hips and back.*

Shortly, we'll take a look through the most common stressors for the hips and lower back. As with previous chapters we'll go through any potential hints and tips to avoid discomfort from these issues. But I feel the glute tensing to stand up straight gets a special mention as it makes such a difference to so many people. The fact that we're mentioning glute strength as being so influential to stability for the second time does hint again at the importance of this muscle group and this will become even clearer as the chapter progresses.

As with previous chapters, the list of influential muscles on the hip and lower back isn't an all-encompassing list of every muscle that can play a part but hopefully it will provide a reference point and will show you enough detail about those I consider to be the most significant.

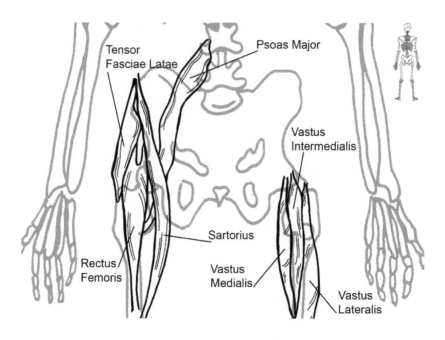

Image 7 – anterior hips and lower back

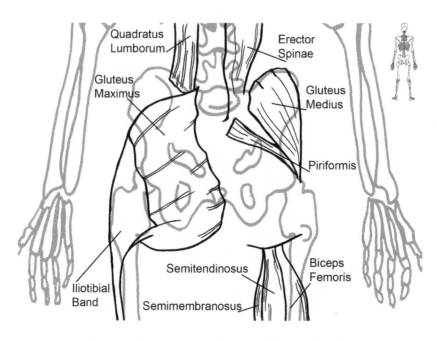

Image 8 – posterior hips and lower back

Common challenges

With most of the areas we've covered so far we've found the predominant challenge faced to be the battle for balance between anterior and posterior muscle groups. However, with the hips and lower back, we also have to consider the battle for balance between left and right. Both of these battles interact with each other so we're left with a constant challenge of trying to maintain equilibrium in the anterior versus posterior chain as well as the left versus right chain (as per the square see-saw analogy). This list is in no particular order or priority but these are the most common causes (not symptoms) of hip and lower back pain that I see:

- standing incorrectly
- sitting incorrectly (sofa, desk/work setup etc.)
- driving
- some exercises/sports (especially those where you're predominantly right or left-handed or right or left-footed)
- looking after a new born baby/children
- gardening/DIY
- household chores
- dog walking
- sleeping.

Standing incorrectly

We've already highlighted the significance of this but addressing and making improvements in your standing position can lead to massive results. If you're consistently standing with your pelvis out of alignment then this can only add to the stress on your hips and lower back. Some people stand really leaning on one hip, others cross one leg over the other and lean while others may have a more subtle lean where they slightly favour one side. If you imagine that you're stood on pressure pads that tell you how much weight you're putting through each foot you should be aiming for 50/50 pressure. You want to be putting equal weight through both your legs to encourage a neutral, balanced pelvis position. This in turn reduces stress on the hips and lower back as you have a neutral, solid base to work from. It must be noted here that there are times when you do have to put more weight through one side over the other due to an injury (for example if you have twisted your right ankle then in the initial short term you would walk with a limp and favour the left leg). However, assuming there isn't a significant injury stopping you from doing so, you should always aim to stand up straight. As we said earlier most people aren't even aware that they lean as it's often a subconscious habit that doesn't cause any pain. Some people even say it feels comfortable to lean on one leg.

There are numerous factors that contribute to a person leaning. We've already referenced the need to do it if there has been an injury but often people will continue to do it long after the injury has healed. I've seen so many people that have had injuries 10, 20 or even 30 or more years ago, injuries that are completely healed now but which would have been responsible for initiating the protective mechanism of leaning. As we frequently mention the body is amazing at firefighting but also likes to get into habits. So once the habit of leaning on one leg has been ingrained, even if we don't need to do it anymore to protect any injuries, it can be a hard habit to crack. Another factor that helps to reinforce the habit is the fact the body like's to mirror other people's body language. We have mirror neurons in our brain that help us to learn through imitation while being essential for our social connections. So it's easy to find yourself leaning without even knowing it simply because the person you're talking to is doing it.

Sometimes, especially if you're standing for a prolonged period of time, you may not have enough strength and endurance in your glutes to keep you stabilised so the body will resort to leaning on one leg for a break. This 'break' while giving the glutes a rest, unintentionally adds more stress to your hips and lower back as you are then out of balance. Another significant contributing factor is carrying children. When I ask clients to think about how they either used to, or currently, carry their children there is often a lightbulb moment where they realise that they've spent months, probably years, carrying a child on one hip over the other. They'll often say that they can picture themselves always carrying them on their right or left hip.

Hopefully, you can see from this selection that there are numerous reasons why you might find that you lean on one leg over the other or favour one side over the other. Many of these reasons can also interlink whereby one factor reinforces another and the habit becomes even harder to break. I can't overstate enough the importance of trying to stand straight and maintain that neutral centre of gravity.

Tip:

- While standing try periodically tensing your glutes for two to three seconds to 'reset' your alignment and ensure that you are neutral and balanced.

Sitting incorrectly (sofa, desk/work setup etc.)

Rather than doing individual sections for sitting on the sofa or sitting at your desk we're just going to group most sitting activities into one section here. The key to it all, similar to when standing, is to keep your alignment neutral. The biggest challenge to that is crossing your legs. This is another challenging one as, like leaning when we're standing, most of us aren't consciously aware of crossing our legs because its's generally comfortable when doing do it. Crossing your legs comes in many forms. It could be just crossing your ankles; it could be sitting with one leg crossed over the other or it could be sitting with one foot tucked underneath you but whatever it is it will mean that your pelvis isn't balanced and neutral. I'm not really sure why we do it but my best guess is that it's the body following the path of least resistance. What I mean by that is that if a muscle is already short then it will be happy being shortened when you're sat. If I have a client who leans on their right leg (which would usually suggest a short right hamstring and short left hip flexor) and I ask them to show me how they sit normally they will usually sit in some way that keeps the left hip flexor shorter (crossing the left ankle over the right or sitting with their left foot tucked underneath them for example). I don't think that this is coincidence and is yet another example of how something like sitting isn't the direct cause of any issues but it can accidentally reinforce your imbalances. Although it's not technically sitting the same can be said for lying on the sofa. Do you usually lie with the same foot crossed over the other or with the same leg bent or hitched out to the side? Although subtle and usually pain-free, all these little actions can help to maintain imbalance and reinforce existing issues. Another way we can 'tilt' is by leaning on an arm rest, be it the arm of the sofa, or your work chair, or any place where you could sit slightly at an angle by accident. Do you always sit in the same spot on the sofa or always lean on one arm rest over the other at work? If you do then you're accidentally lengthening one side of your lower back and shortening the other and potentially increasing the stress on your lower back by not being neutral.

Tips:

- Try to mix up where you sit on the sofa to make sure you're not always sat at the same angle.
- Try to avoid crossing your feet or legs when you are sat and sit equally on each glute (similar to the pressure pads on the feet, try and imagine you have to sit with 50/50 weight distribution).

Driving

Although driving requires sitting, so all of the last section is applicable here, there are also a couple of driving specific challenges I want to mention. Again, if driving is to be a factor, it's often due to the repetitive nature of lots of little actions that take an effect and the potential of prolonged sitting in an incorrect position. Driving also takes many forms here. At one end of the scale we have people who do a lot of motorway driving. The main challenges here can be the right hip flexor shortening from regularly holding the foot on the accelerator and also the potential of hitching the left leg up and resting it against the centre console due to the infrequent need for gear changes (this is based on a right-hand drive car so swap it round if your car is left-hand drive). The same challenges can also apply to those driving automatic cars as gear changes aren't required. Moving to the other end of the scale we've got taxi drivers or delivery drivers doing lots of short, sharp journeys around town that include lots of gear changes. Here, the potential is there for the left hip flexor to shorten if there's lots of hovering over the clutch and lots of left leg usage. So, you can see that even under the umbrella of driving there can be different challenges depending on what your driving entails.

Another factor that I've seen regularly over the years is people's seat being too low and therefore their hips being flexed more than they need to be (i.e. their hip angle is less than 90 degrees) which can lead to shorter hip flexors. For many clients raising their seat so that they sit at 90 degrees, or as close to this as possible, has made a massive difference on their hips and lower back. Likewise, ensuring that the seat back is at the correct angle to actually support you (again, I'd recommend as upright and close to 90 degrees as possible) rather than tilted back too far, can have similarly significant effects.

Finally, I've seen many clients over the years who have, it turns out, been sat too close to the wheel and have therefore had their hips flexed too much unnecessarily. Although it's another simple fix, being sat at the correct distance from the steering wheel can have a significant impact on balance and pelvic position. Each contributing factor is significant in its own right but worst case scenario putting all the factors together, you could see how if you had a poor seat angle, were sat too close to the wheel, were leaning down on the centre console and resting your left leg against the centre console, the act of driving could have a monumental impact on your hips and lower back.

Tips:

- Take regular breaks from driving to make sure you're not 'fixed' in the same position for too long.
- Make sure you're not hitching up your hip.
- Make sure that you are not sat too close to the steering wheel.
- Make sure your seat back is positioned at the right angle and is supporting you.
- Make sure that your seat is not too low and causing you to flex your hips unnecessarily.

Some exercises/sports (especially those where you're predominantly right or left-handed or right or left-footed)

If you're doing any exercises or sports out of neutral alignment for long enough, at a high enough intensity or a combination of both, then eventually the lower back and hips will have something to say about it. We'll cover some of the more obvious examples first, activities where you are forced into positions of misalignment simply by doing the activity. We'll then cover some of the less obvious activities that we often think of as being good for our backs and hips but which can catch us out if we're not doing them correctly. Any sport where we rotate to one side more than the other will inevitably cause muscular imbalance, whether that's throwing, kicking, any racket sport, golf, cricket (batting or bowling), football, rugby, netball, boxing, kickboxing – the list is endless. This doesn't mean that these sports are all dangerous for us but we have to recognise that they aren't neutral and we may have to stretch or strengthen accordingly to counterbalance the potential effects of the sport. It's also about remembering what's being shortened and what's being lengthened. For example, if you're right-handed and the right side of your lower back aches after a game of tennis then it's likely to be overstretched (think of the stretch of the right side through a serve or a forehand shot), so stretching it after would make it worse.

If we're misaligned then the chances are that the piriformis and iliotibial band (IT band) on one leg will be shorter and tighter than the other. Therefore, activities that we would think of as equal such as horse riding or breaststroke swimming, which involve movements that laterally rotate the hip (requiring the piriformis and IT band to shorten) could accidentally be shortening them further and adding more stress to the hips and lower back. Likewise, referring back to the square see-saw analogy, most people often have tightness in opposite hip flexors and hamstrings that are counterbalancing each other. Therefore, activities that you may think are strengthening your core (e.g. sit-ups, planks, squats and deadlifts) could actually be reinforcing the underlying imbalances. It's important to highlight here that I think sit-ups are rubbish and do more harm than good. In terms of balance, all they do is shorten up the anterior chain (hip flexors and abdominals) which increases the potential to cause stress to your lower back. Say you are out of balance; sit-ups will just tighten up the already tight hip flexor. I've lost count of how many clients have come in with back pain who had started doing more sit-ups in the weeks leading up to the onset of their back pain. They do nothing for your glutes, which I believe are the most important muscles in stabilising the pelvis, apart from slightly overstretching them as well. So back pain or not, don't do sit-ups! Now planks I love but you need to be in a good enough place in the first place for them to complement you. If you are significantly out of balance then even they have the potential to irritate and exacerbate any imbalance further. We're aiming for a nice 50/50 balance between left and right but if you're out of balance, say 55/45, then when you squat or deadlift you'll be doing those activities with that imbalance. So, you may be inadvertently dropping down slightly on one hip more than the other or driving up through with one glute more than the other. Again, although these activities are great for you if you are equal enough and strong enough initially, they can work against you and accidentally reinforce your imbalances if you're not.

Running gets its own section in the upcoming chapters but here gets a small mention. Just thinking of the forces at play (up to seven times your body weight going through your joints when you run) if those forces aren't being spread evenly then you can see how eventually the stress can build up. Running is generally a repetitive action with few, if any, short, sharp, surprise movements. However, where it is repetitive and, in some cases, relentless (longer distance running) any underlying imbalances tend to get found out over time. I can't remember many clients actually having their back spasm while running but many will come to me saying that their hip or back pain has gradually worsened over the previous weeks/months and that they don't remember any injury occurring or doing anything that could have started it all off. That's the issue right there though because there wouldn't have been an initial injury at all, it's just that running has gradually reinforced their imbalances (tight muscles get tighter, overstretched muscles get more overstretched) until they'd reached a point where it was too uncomfortable to carry on and they sought help. This is yet another example of how the body will try its best to adapt but will, eventually, reach a tipping point where you start to feel pain.

Tips:

- If your sport or activity encourages you to work out of balance then you may need to stretch and strengthen accordingly to counteract that imbalance.
- Don't do sit-ups!
- Seek advice or treatment if you feel you may be out of balance. You may well save yourself a lot of time and discomfort by addressing the imbalance in the initial stages.

Looking after a new born baby/children

We've already mentioned the potential challenge posed by carrying a child on one hip over the other. We won't go over the same things again but it is so important to try and swap arms and, ideally, spend as much time in a neutral standing position as possible. The realities of this are very tricky as you don't get to spend much time in a neutral position with children so just trying to alternate which arm you hold them with is probably the more realistic target here. They get bigger and wriggle more so the challenge only gets tougher but if you can balance out the stress, as best you can, as opposed to always putting the stress through one hip or one side of your lower back it can make a world of difference. In the initial stages there can be a lot of sitting down with the baby and this links into the earlier challenge of trying to sit as neutrally as possible. If you always sit in the same spot on the sofa to cuddle the baby and your position isn't neutral, the prolonged incorrect sitting compounded over weeks and months could eventually lead to hip and lower back discomfort. Similarly, you may always lay down on one side when playing with the child on the floor. Doing this once isn't an issue but if it's repeated week after week, alongside other compounding factors it could easily become a significant factor in contributing to pain further down the line. Over the years, a handful of clients have noticed that they really struggled with being bent over and holding their child's hands when they're learning to walk. This would be a hard activity to adapt but the key is to not stretch out the already overstretched lower back if it does ache.

Tips:

- Really make a conscious effort to make sure you're not carrying the child on one hip more than the other.
- Try to vary your positions when sitting with the child so that you don't accidentally repeatedly sit in a poor, unbalanced position.

  I think this a good place to remind ourselves that the body is resilient and adaptable and that we can't be in position A at all times – it's just not realistic. However, this is all about us trying to avoid continual repetition of incorrect positions and thus avoiding pain and avoiding making pain worse by doing the incorrect actions in an attempt to relieve the pain.

Gardening/DIY

I could write a whole book just about the challenges faced in gardening and DIY and the links to lower back and hip issues but we're just going to cover the most common challenges.

The first factor, which applies to many gardening/DIY activities is the fact it's rare that we're ever leaning backwards. If we think of performing activities such as digging, lifting, painting, sawing, drilling, planting flowers and cutting hedges it's rare that we'd find ourselves leaning backwards. Herein lies the potential for the overstretched area to complain again. Other activities may not stretch your lower back as much but still require you to do an activity with your arms out in front of you. I've lost count of the number of clients who've suffered a day or two after mowing the lawn, or raking leaves or sweeping because they're repetitive movements where you're slightly flexed forwards, reaching out in front of you and slightly overstretching your back for potentially extended periods of time. Some people feel the urge to straighten up and lean backwards after activities like this (good) while others will feel their back is stiff and 'tight' as a result and will try to stretch it out further by trying to touch their toes or by twisting or bending side to side to 'free it up' (bad). Linking back to the challenge of standing neutrally some of these activities can be done while accidentally leaning on one leg more than the other (e.g. painting or rolling). Similarly, if the job requires moving things out the way then are we lifting things properly or quickly? Do you get immediate pain if you lift something incorrectly, taking more weight on one side or twisting when you pick something up? Probably not the first time. But if you spend a few hours digging (leaning forward and twisting to one side more than the other) and then plant some flowers (leaning forward and probably twisting one side more than the other) then it's the cumulative effects of the repetitive stretching that could take their toll in the end. Usually, the pain comes the next day when you do something trivial like reach to pick the kettle up or to put your shoes on and it's then that the already tired, overstretched and grumpy lower back decides it wants a break and can't be stretched anymore and stops you in your tracks.

Tips:

- If you've got to lift something try and lift equally and properly – don't pivot from your back.
- Take regular breaks to make sure you're not repeating the same movement for extended periods of time.

Household chores

At first glance this may seem like a bit of an odd one but I've seen so many different examples of seemingly simple household activities either contributing towards, or being the tipping point for, back pain that it needs its own section.

Let's start with ironing. It wouldn't be seen by many as a danger sport but when you think about the functional mechanics of it, although there are few dramatic or extreme movements involved, you have to stand slightly leaning forward for a prolonged period of time which means the lower back is slightly overstretched the whole time. As we know overstretched muscles are most likely to complain, so this isn't a great position for the lower back full stop but factor in leaning on or favouring one leg while ironing as well and the stress to the back gets magnified even more.

Washing up can put very similar stresses on the lower back and, likewise, these stresses can also be exacerbated further if you lean on one leg while doing this. If you're thinking that doesn't apply to you because you've got a dishwasher then you're partly right but I'm afraid using a dishwasher comes with a different set of challenges. Loading and unloading a dishwasher is something we often do without thinking about, sometimes overstretching, possibly while leaning on one leg and don't get any pain while doing it. But it's for those very reasons that so many clients have hurt themselves when this has proven to be the tipping point to highlighting an underlying imbalance.

Vacuuming is another one where it's seemingly innocuous but it's easy to accidentally overstretch while reaching, leaning forward, or trying to get to an awkward spot or when grabbing the vacuum to take it up or down stairs. I'm sure you can think of other similar activities along these lines and, as always, I'm not trying to make you overthink everything you do but it's often minor changes that lead to the biggest results so if you can do a few activities in a slightly better position it can only have positive effects.

Tips:

- Try to break up chores to make sure you're not fixed in one position for too long.
- If you are stood for a long time make sure you're standing equally balanced on each leg.

Dog walking

This might also seem an odd one at first glance but it's also come up too many times with clients not to mention it.

Firstly, even before you've left the house, you've got to get the lead on the dog. Bending down to put a dog's lead on is a classic example of where the lower back reaches a tipping point and decides that it can't be stretched anymore, leading to a spasm. It's an action you've done hundreds of times before without thinking about it but it can be done easily and quickly and if done at slightly the wrong angle it can cause enough of a stress to cause a spasm. Spasms aside it is an action that you may do hundreds of times so it's important to try and do it as equally as possible.

The next potential challenge comes with the factor of usually walking the dog on the same side, holding the lead in one hand more frequently and the potential risk of being pulled or twisted on one side over the other. I've seen many clients where they had an underlying imbalance that they weren't aware of until their dog pulling them one way caused them to have pain. This was actually the tipping point because that area was already overstretched but they didn't know.

A final factor can be if you regularly walk your dog on the same route. A lot of the time we're walking on a surface that has a slight camber that we are not even aware of (pavement, promenade, sand, woodland) because our body is always adapting to keep us upright. However, if we always walk the same way and follow the same cambers we can inadvertently be causing, or more likely reinforcing, pelvic imbalances. For example, promenades often lean slightly towards the sea so if you always walk the same way on a promenade then one hip will be dropping slightly towards the sea. Pavements in residential areas often have dropped kerbs so say you always walk the same loop with the dog then you'll always be walking on the same pavements with the same drops.

Tips:

- Make sure you're bending down slowly and concentrating when you're putting the lead on the dog.
- Make sure you mix up your routes to ensure you're getting variety underfoot.
- If you can and the dog will cooperate, try to chop and change the hand you hold the lead in.

Sleeping

Hopefully, this section might save you a bit of money. I'd say about 50% of clients with back pain will tell me in their initial assessment session that their mattress is rubbish and is probably a big cause of their back pain. Although a nice new mattress does often feel great it doesn't change your body. If you're rubbish at driving and you buy a faster car you're still rubbish at driving. Likewise, if you are misaligned and spend £2,000 on a new mattress then you're still misaligned.

However supportive a mattress is, it can only support you and your alignment. It doesn't matter how much you spend it won't provide a magic cure. I've often seen clients who have bought a new mattress and their back pain has worsened as a result. Once they realise that buying a firmer, more supportive mattress has simply highlighted their imbalances more they aren't often that happy. By working on the cause and not the symptom they feel the benefits of the more supportive mattress once they're in a more neutral alignment but this often happens a few weeks later than the instant result for which they were hoping. I say the same to everyone – make sure you're the best you can be before getting a new mattress. If your hip flexors on one leg are tighter than the other side for example, you're more likely to hitch that leg up when you're asleep and therefore potentially maintain the imbalance in the pelvis when you're resting. If you can work on getting to a place where you're neutral before going to bed then you've got a better chance of sleeping neutrally, getting maximum rest and repair and therefore feeling better in the morning. People with chronic back pain will often struggle most first thing in the morning because they've likely just spent hours accidentally reinforcing the fact that they're out of balance and accidentally stressing muscles while sleeping.

Tip:

- Don't spend loads on a mattress and hope it's the miracle cure. Get your body into the best alignment you can through stretching and strengthening and you'll get the most benefit out of sleeping.

Sciatica

As per the previous chapters some issues get their own section and sciatica is one of those. In my opinion, this is another term that is thrown around far too often. You don't have to do much searching online before you could quickly panic yourself into believing you have a defective spine. Sciatica refers to the irritation of the sciatic nerve, a nerve which originates at the lower back and branches out and runs all the way down the leg into the foot.

Like we said, if you search for information on sciatica, near enough all of it will point you towards a spinal issue, yet most people are diagnosed without any scans on their back to ascertain whether there is a spinal issue. If you dig deep enough though you can occasionally find some information mentioning the piriformis muscle as a potential cause. The piriformis is a deep muscle underneath your glutes. The sciatic nerve usually runs underneath the piriformis but in some cases it runs through it. Either way, if the piriformis is overworking, which is almost a guarantee if your glutes aren't strong enough, then it will enlarge and become inflamed due to the extra workload. Eventually, usually over a long-term period of many months or years, it can get so large and inflamed that it will then press against the sciatic nerve. At this point the classic symptoms of pain deep in the buttock, or nerve pain down the hamstring/back of the leg, or nerve pain into the heel or, if you're unlucky, a combination of all of the symptoms will start to develop. Where the piriformis is the cause of the issue it's termed piriformis syndrome. As someone who doesn't like to diagnose and create potentially unnecessary stress, I will often tell clients that they have sciatic nerve irritation. I am aware I that don't have any scanning equipment available at my practice to confirm this for sure but I strongly believe that the vast majority of people are suffering from sciatic nerve irritation due to the piriformis compressing the nerve. I base this on a few factors. Firstly, I've never seen a client with sciatic nerve pain where the piriformis isn't tight and inflamed. Secondly, if the piriformis were fine on both sides then that would indicate a balanced and neutral pelvis. If this were the case then you could argue that the only cause of the sciatic nerve stress would have to come from the lower back. In over a decade of working and seeing hundreds of different clients, I have never once seen this. Every single client I have seen with sciatic nerve irritation has had an imbalance in their pelvis and a tight piriformis on the side that they are experiencing the sciatic nerve symptoms. In a typical treatment session for this issue I would spend a few minutes working on the clients lower back as undoubtedly there would be an imbalance there as well and there would be some discomfort. However, when I start to work on the affected tight piriformis, always after doing one minute on the other side before to show the client the difference when a piriformis isn't tight and inflamed, nearly every time just light work on the piriformis recreates some or all of the symptoms that the client is experiencing. This, for both of us, confirms that this is the source of the irritation as we can essentially recreate the symptom.

I believe and have numerous clients that provide proof, that through a combination of treatment, stretches and glute strengthening you can get to a more neutral pelvic position. This stops the piriformis from compressing the sciatic nerve and allows you to get back to being pain-free once again. It isn't often a quick process as it does usually, as previously mentioned, take months or years of piriformis overuse to get to a point where it compresses the nerve so, whoever you see, don't expect any quick miracle cure.

It all comes back to alignment and balance. Often, steroid injections and painkillers are recommended and clients are told that the pain will go away by itself in a few weeks. If you have been out of alignment for months and develop sciatic nerve irritation then taking painkillers or having an injection isn't going to get you realigned. You may get some temporary relief but you're only firefighting and not getting to the root cause. Another common recommendation to 'assist' with recovery is to do stretches that stretch the sciatic nerve. The nerve is already under stress from being compressed so I can't see how adding more stress to an already stressed area is going to help. Clients who have been separately advised to do this nearly always tell me they think it might have made things worse or in the best case scenario, it did nothing.

One final important note here though is that sciatic nerve irritation would usually only affect one side. Therefore, if numbness or nerve sensations are being felt on both sides equally then this could be a sign of something more significant and you should seek medical advice promptly.

Hip replacement surgery

Although medical and technological advancements mean that both recovery and success rates for hip replacement surgery are improving all the time it is still an invasive procedure and, as with any operation, carries an element of risk. As per any procedure I would always encourage you to explore all options before committing to an operation. However, if that is the last option available to you then there are a couple of tips that I'd like to share. If you are lined up for surgery, say in a few months' time, it's important to be as strong as you can beforehand. Pain allowing, the more strength you have in and around the hip before the surgery the better your recovery will be afterwards. I think some people, though I can understand why, just wait for their surgery thinking that there's no point doing anything before as it could make it worse and they're having surgery anyway so what's the point. It is obvious to say the surgery itself is a massive part of the process but how successful your operation turns out to be is massively linked to the work you put in to strengthening all the muscles around the joint. I'm a firm believer that this process starts before the surgery not just after. By stimulating the muscles you're preparing them for the road to recovery after the operation. You can have a successful operation and see X-rays that confirm that the joint is as it should be and that's a fantastic start but if all the surrounding structures around the hip aren't strong enough to support this new, functional hip joint then you'll never get to fully reap the benefits. Understandably, there is a lot of emphasis on post-operative rehabilitation exercises and rightly so but I just think it's important that, if the situation allows, that you make a start before the surgery begins.

Now let's say the operation has gone well, you've been given the exercises for the hip strengthening and you're ready to start the hard work. The next tip I've got, although adding to your workload initially, could well be a game changer to your future. Here it is – don't forget your other leg. We mentioned earlier in the chapter that there are occasions when we have to favour one leg over the other and early recovery after hip replacement surgery definitely qualifies as one of those occasions. In the initial stages you have to put more weight through your other leg and that's that. However, as much as the majority of the focus for rehabilitation does need to be on the operated hip, you do have to consider that the other leg will be working harder to support you so will also need attention. I've only seen a few clients myself but have heard of many, many more, who have ended up needing the opposite hip, knee or ankle operated on a few years down the line. Granted, in some circumstances, it has been due to the initial operation not being as successful as hoped for meaning that the individual has had to carry on putting more weight through their other leg to manage the discomfort, which has eventually taken its toll. Unfortunately, although in most cases the operation was successful, all the post-operative rehabilitation was focussed solely on the hip that was operated on. This focus meant that, even though the surgery was successful, the body had continued to favour the other leg as a habit and eventually this continued imbalance had taken its toll on the other, previously fine hip. That's why I'm so passionate about reminding people that the body gets into habits quickly and easily and won't break them by itself. Just because your surgically repaired hip is fine the body won't automatically put you back to the middle – it takes a conscious effort.

I feel that numerous secondary operations could be avoided if the focus were put on to the body as a whole not just on the hip that was operated on. I've also seen this pattern repeated a lot with knee and ankle surgery. Luckily there have been a number of clients where we've been able to break the cycle and, I feel, avoid further procedures. So often I've heard stories like,

> I had my right hip operated on three years ago and it's completely fine. I'm so much happier with it, it doesn't give me problems anymore and that's not why I'm here. I'm here because my left knee has gradually been getting worse the last few months and now I'm struggling to walk without a limp.

I've seen numerous examples of this principle in action with some combination of hip, knee, ankle or Achilles' tendon, where an operation on one leg is the catalyst for pain on the other leg years down the line. So, in short, remember your other leg and don't solely focus on the repaired hip. You don't want all the time and effort you've put in to building up your strength, stability and function for your hip to have to be repeated again for the opposite hip five years down the line.

Degenerative disc disease/spinal discopathy/bulging, herniated and slipped discs

We discussed this in great detail in the neck and upper back chapter so I won't repeat it all again here. However, although most of the information is transferrable to the lower spine, we can still tailor a couple of points to the lower back and hips. We briefly mentioned the introduction of upright scanning and, as I said, I think it is a step in the right direction as the fact that you're weight-bearing at the time of the scan can give a slightly truer representation of the stresses on your spine compared to being laid flat on your back. However, if one of the biggest contributors happened to be the glutes being weaker on one side over the other side then standing up straight for a scan may still hide the biggest contributing factor.

In the last chapter I got you to visualise the spinal column as perfectly neutral until we added a wonky skull to the top. The equivalent for the lower body would be having a rotated pelvis at the bottom of the spine. In the same way that the upper spine has to counteract the skull position, the lower spine has to do the same to counteract the pelvic position. Let's visualise a rotated pelvis that's rotated down to the back right (short right hamstrings) and to the front left (short left hip flexors). If the spine didn't counteract this twist, it would be pulled over to the right. So, the muscles of the lower back shorten on the left to realign the spine but this means that the disc could potentially bulge out or get pinched because the vertebrae aren't stacked neutrally on top of each other again. As always alignment is key, so if you are able to stretch and strengthen your way into a neutral position then you can see how this helps to create the neutral spine that we are all aiming for. The flipside to this is that it's equally as easy to see how back and neck pain can occur if the spine is relentlessly having to fight against lower and upper spine misalignment due to imbalance and dysfunction.

General tips

Hopefully, you'll have noticed a few common themes throughout this chapter but let's recap. Primarily it's all about balance. I keep going back to the square see-saw analogy but I think it's the best way to visualise how you need to maintain that equilibrium. You may have also heard the pelvis described before as a bowl that's full and that you don't want it to tip too far in any direction. So, when you're stood, really try and concentrate on standing equally with a 50/50 spread of your weight through each leg. If you find yourself leaning then tensing your glutes equally for just a couple of seconds is often enough to 'reset' and get you back to neutral. If you find you're struggling with this (either you can't get your glutes to fire up or you feel like one side is working much more than the other) then this could be an indicator that there's improvements to be made so I'd recommend exploring getting assessed by a professional to create a plan to make you stronger and more neutral. Reinforcing the neutral theme, think about trying to sit as neutrally as you can. Yes, you'll slump sometimes and probably cross your legs or ankles occasionally (I know I still do and I've been doing this for years) but the quicker and more often you catch yourself and 'reset' the fewer issues sitting is likely to give you.

A more general tip for the body as a whole, not just the lower back and hips, is if you've got stuff to carry that should take two trips but that you could probably squeeze in to one if you loaded yourself up, just take two trips. A minute saved here and there pails into insignificance if you reach that tipping point, have a back spasm and can't sit, stand or walk pain-free for a week. We are all guilty of doing it occasionally but if you are always rushing and carrying more than you should then eventually the body will find a way to slow you down. Tied in with that is the use of a proper lifting technique when we do need to lift something. It's more than a little idealistic to aim for a perfectly straight back with perfect knee and hip form every single time we pick something up but if it's in your conscious awareness more often than not then you're much less likely to overstretch your lower back by accident when reaching for something.

What not to do

If it hurts don't stretch it. If your lower back hurts don't stretch it. It's probably overstretched from a tight hamstring and/or piriformis. If your groin/adductor area feels sore then don't stretch it. It's probably overstretched due to a tight piriformis and IT band. If your hip flexor is sore don't stretch it. The chances are the hamstrings on the same side are short and tight and therefore the hip flexor is overstretched. The same goes for a sore hamstring as the chances are the hip flexors are tighter on the same side. I'm sure you get the theme of this by now but it's never a bad time to reinforce it. As we said earlier, if your sciatic nerve is being irritated then don't stretch it and add even more stress to it. I also strongly recommend against targeted lower back strengthening unless you have been advised by a professional for a very specific reason. Lower backs are usually under enough stress already and I've seen so many times how trying to strengthen them has become the tipping point for pain or injury. Finally, a great way to avoid lower back stress is to avoid sit-ups – they're not worth the risk.

What to do

Hamstring, piriformis and hip flexor stretching are key to achieving and maintaining as neutral a pelvis position as possible. However, for most achieving this neutrality may well require stretching the muscles in different ratios initially. If you have a typical imbalance and say, for example, you have tight left hip flexors and tight right hamstrings and piriformis then you may well need to do more stretches on those than the same muscles on the opposite side. I would always advise you see someone professionally rather than make up your own ratios but I often have clients who periodically or permanently need to stretch at a 2:1 or 3:2 ratio, whereby they will stretch one side more than the other. If you're out of balance and stretch both sides equally you may improve your flexibility slightly but you won't make any changes to your imbalance which is the most probable cause of back and hip pain.

In terms of strengthening a lot depends on how well aligned you are in the first place. Glute strengthening is key so if you were relatively equal then activities including squats, lunges and single leg dead lifts would be great to build upon the existing strength. However, if you're significantly out of alignment then these exercises might be too difficult or you may be inadvertently doing them incorrectly. The same goes for planks. If you're strong enough then planks and all the associated variations of them, are a fantastic way of maintaining strength and balance. However, if you're too weak or misaligned then they can add further stress to your underlying imbalances. If in doubt seek advice from a professional who can gauge where you're starting from and set you off on the right path to increased strength and balance.

Foam rollers are also of great use both in terms of the physical benefits of rolling the muscles as well as their potential use as a diagnostic tool for self-analysis. For example, if you were using the roller on your calves and one was more painful than the other, this could be a sign that one leg is working harder than the other and you may be out of balance. Saying that, as we know, we do many activities that are out of balance (so in this scenario you could be right-footed and have just finished playing football so you would probably expect your right calf to be more tired) so don't panic every time there is a slight difference on the roller. But if you see a continual pattern (maybe one calf is always more tender after you run) then this could be an indicator of imbalances in the network. Personally, I think that foam rollers are not only especially effective on the calves and IT band but also do a good job on the quadriceps (quads), glutes and hamstrings. At the moment you can get smooth rollers or harder ones with nodules on or handheld massage sticks (who knows what the future holds) so through trial and error I encourage you to find what you like. Some people think the smooth rollers don't offer enough resistance while others say the harder rollers are too painful so play around and see which one, or combination of rollers, suits you best.

Other factors

Like the neck there can also be issues with lower backs that are neurological in nature and, again, issues such as bone spurs, damaged vertebrae or stress fractures can all be factors. However, you should remember that just because you have been diagnosed with one of these issues doesn't mean that improvements can't still be made. Altering your training or activity levels, as well as ensuring you are as balanced as possible, can quickly reduce the stress. Labral tears are another issue where improvements can be made, in many cases without the need for surgery, although it may be necessary in some cases. Finally, we covered a lot of the physiological realities of whiplash in the chapter on the neck and shoulders but the characteristics are the same further down the body and can easily affect the lower back just as much as the neck after an accident.

CHAPTER 7

Knees

Just like everything else we've covered so far, knees are complicated. Although knees may not be subjected to as broad a range of movement as other joints they are still susceptible to a variety of stresses and strains. This is quite an extreme example but think about the forces that must go through the knee when someone is completing a triple jump. Sprinting, in its own right, asks so many questions of the knee joint before you even get to the skips and then finish in a crumpled heap with the landing. I know for most people it's not your everyday activity and not something I'd advocate trying without experience but it's a fascinating example showing the types of forces that can be tolerated through the knee joint.

As we know joints can only tolerate what they can by relying on the function of the supporting structures surrounding them. Although we mainly think of the knee as flexing and extending it can also slightly internally and externally rotate. Therefore, all the muscles, ligaments and tendons above, below and surrounding the knee need to be working in harmony to stabilise and control the joint through all the capable movements. It's no wonder then that knee pain is so common as there are so many points in the network where stress can occur. It only takes the quads and hamstrings to be out of balance, or the muscles of the shin to be out of balance with the calves, for stress to be felt at the knee. Above the knee it's not just the quads and hamstrings that need to be working in harmony. For example, if the lateral upper leg (the abductors) are dominating over the medial upper leg (the adductors), or vice versa, then this would cause the upper leg to rotate slightly externally or internally. This in turn would put stress on the knee joint as it would be functioning out of neutral alignment. This repeated stress can have a negative impact on the patella and the patella tendon if it isn't tracking neutrally. Likewise, the ligaments on the inside and outside of the knee (medial and lateral collateral ligaments), as well as the deep ligaments at the front and back of the knee (anterior and posterior cruciate ligaments), are susceptible to stress and potential injury if the joint is consistently misaligned. However, it's not all doom and gloom as the correct stretching and strengthening can usually sort out these functional imbalances.

Looking above the knee it's crucial that the glutes are strong and equal (any excuse to drop in the standing up straight and equally tip again). This ensures that the hamstrings don't shorten up and therefore the quads don't become overstretched. This also ensures that the IT band doesn't shorten and therefore the adductors don't become overstretched. A short, tight IT band is what leads to the condition of 'runner's knee' but we'll cover that in more detail later.

Looking below the knee again it's crucial that the ankle joint is stable and neutral so that the muscles of the shin (dorsiflexors) and the muscles of the calf (plantar flexors) can work equally. Interestingly, ankle stability isn't solely based on ankle strength and it is significantly impacted by alignment further up the network in the glutes and hips but we'll cover that further in the next chapter.

Sometimes with knee injuries you simply get unlucky. It's not uncommon for elite athletes especially but also us normal folk, to suffer anterior cruciate ligament (ACL) injuries because their foot is planted when the force is applied against them and the ACL just snaps. All the alignment and strengthening in the world can't stop some injuries from happening. However, there are plenty of knee injuries that occur from seemingly innocuous actions, such as twisting or landing on one leg, where no one else is around and no other forces are at play. Here, the body just reaches that tipping point again and often there is no obvious warning. The key word from that last sentence is obvious because it may well be that the knee has been functioning out of alignment for weeks, months or maybe even years without the person knowing. But therein lies the benefit of stretching and strengthening (and treatment) because you reduce the chances of becoming misaligned and, as such, greatly reduce your risks of getting injured.

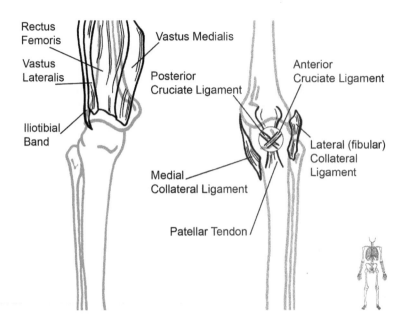

Image 9 – anterior knee

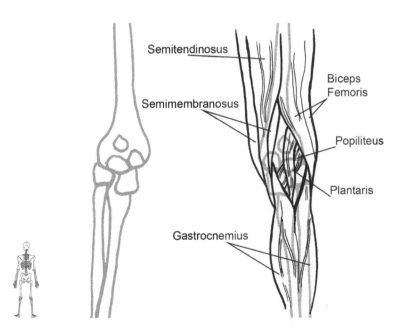

Image 10 – posterior knee

Common Challenges

Below are the most common challenges for the knees that I've seen regularly over the years. They cover issues of alignment, functionality, stability and others. I've found that, as with the areas we've already covered, there isn't one consistent challenge for the knee but often a myriad of factors at play in a number of varying situations. As always, this list won't cover every cause of every single knee issue I've ever seen but it covers the vast majority:

- standing incorrectly (including gardening, DIY and household chores)
- sitting incorrectly (sofa, desk/work setup etc.)
- driving
- running
- some exercises/sports (including those where you're predominantly right or left-footed)
- sleeping

Standing incorrectly (including gardening, DIY and household chores)

Most of what we could talk about here we have already covered in the last chapter on hips and lower back but it is always worth reaffirming the importance of standing up straight and equally. If you stand on leg more than the other then you will be putting more weight through that knee joint than the other knee. As the occasional one-off, or if short-term leaning is required while recovering from another injury, then any effect would be negligible so long as you rebalance soon after. But if this process is repeated day after day, week after week, year after year, then this compounding additional stress on the joint could start to take a toll. More importantly, if you are standing out of balance it also means all the supporting muscles will also be out of balance. When considering the vital role that muscles play on stabilising and supporting joints, it's easy to see how repetitive overuse of some muscles and underuse of others could affect alignment of the knee joint and accelerate the rate of stress on the joint. This point is emphasised in the fact that in over a decade of seeing clients I've never had a client present with equal knee pain. Very occasionally I'll come across a client where both knees hurt but one will always hurt more than the other. More often than not, a client will present with pain in one knee only. Sometimes clients will put the pain down to a recent activity they've just started (often this activity is running) and blame that for the onset of the pain. My reply is always the same – if running were the sole cause of the issue and it was just your body's way of saying it didn't like running, then both knees would hurt the same. Running may well have highlighted an underlying imbalance (we'll cover this more later in the chapter) but it's unlikely to have been the direct cause of the pain.

Although we've digressed away from standing up straight, rightly so because it was an important point, let's come back to it now. If you lean on one leg more than the other, usually this is while you are doing seemingly simple activities, like the washing up or painting a wall, you are putting more pressure through one knee over the other. Even activities where you can't fully lean on one leg, such as being up a ladder, may still be influenced by your imbalance and you may slightly favour one leg over the other so make sure you work on this if it is a factor for you.

Tip:

- Tense those glutes and stand up straight!

Sitting incorrectly (sofa, desk/work setup etc.)

Again, most of what we talked about in the last chapter is relevant here. Whether it's crossing our ankles, crossing our legs, sitting with one foot tucked underneath us, sitting with one leg out to the side or whichever other variation of sitting we do, nothing beats sitting neutrally. As always, though, it's worth remembering we aspire to be neutral as often as we can but we won't be spot on all the time. If you're sat next to someone on the sofa and chatting to them it might be a bit odd if you were sat perfectly with a neutral spine and head position looking forward into the middle of the room, never turning to face them when speaking to them. However, if you're sat watching a film by yourself for two hours with your ankle tucked underneath you and only realise you were doing it when you start to get pins and needles, this is the kind of situation we're aiming to make improvements with. It definitely takes a conscious effort initially to start noticing how you're sitting. You won't get a reminder to do this because you probably won't be in immediate pain if you sit a little off neutral but each time you catch yourself and 'reset' your position it's a win for the body.

Another time where you should keep an eye on your position is while you're doing any DIY or gardening that requires you to kneel or squat down for lengthy periods. You may find that you squat down on one side more than the other or may even squat down with one knee bent and the other leg out straight. If you have any underlying ankle, knee or hip issues that mean you can't squat or kneel down as well on one side due to pain or range of movement restrictions, then it may not be possible for you to squat or kneel down equally (I personally struggle with this due to having a limited range of movement in one of my ankles after an operation.) If this is this case and being equal in your position isn't an option, it's even more imperative than normal that you take more regular breaks to reduce the impact on the knee that's taking more of the load. It's also common for prolonged kneeling to be uncomfortable due to the physical pressure on the knee joint and patella from kneeling, especially on firmer surfaces, so the use of individual knee pads or a moveable kneeling pad can be beneficial.

Tips:
- Try to mix up where you sit on the sofa to make sure you're not always sat at the same angle.
- Try to avoid crossing your feet or legs when you are sat and try to sit equally on each glute.
- Make sure you take regular breaks if you're doing activities that require kneeling or squatting for lengthy periods.

Driving

The potential causes of stress on the knees while driving are pretty much the same as those that cause stress to the hips and lower back but there's no harm in covering them again. Firstly, the seat distance to the pedals is crucial because if we're sat too close then our knees will be flexed more than they need to be. Of course, you don't want to be sat so far away you can barely reach the pedals but I've found that, on the whole, most clients sit a little closer than needed and adjusting the distance slightly does have a positive impact. Secondly, if the seat is too low then that also increases the angle of flexion in the knees and can cause an avoidable stress to the joint. Again, you wouldn't expect to make a drastic change but you may find just a slight increase in the seat height could improve your knee position. Finally, and as we've mentioned before this is more common in motorway driving or those with automatic cars, hitching your left leg up when it's not being used will flex the knee unnecessarily so try to have your left leg out in front of you when driving (this is again based on a right-hand drive car so swap it round if your car is left-hand drive).

Tips:

- Take regular breaks from driving to make sure you're not 'fixed' in the same position for too long.
- Make sure you're not hitching up your knee if you're not using it.
- Check whether you are sat too close to the steering wheel.
- Check whether the seat is too low and making you flex your knees unnecessarily.

<u>Running</u>

Although knee pain and running are often heard in the same sentence (after all, there is an injury called 'runner's knee') they really don't need to be. As I mentioned earlier in the chapter, running is often labelled as a cause of knee pain but I like to think of it slightly differently in terms of it being running simply highlighting your existing imbalance. There is nowhere to hide in running – the whole body has to be on point and working efficiently for running to be beneficial for you. It's easy to see how a slight imbalance, combined with the force of up to seven times your body weight going through your knee, repeated over thousands and thousands of steps could eventually create a larger imbalance and ultimately lead to discomfort. Occasionally, of course, you can slip and twist the knee or stumble and jar the knee on landing and that's often simple bad luck. However, most knee complaints surrounding running build over a period of weeks or usually months and can't be pinpointed back to a specific cause. This links back to the most probable cause being an underlying, often unknown, imbalance that becomes magnified due to the mechanics of running. The last chapter began to highlight the importance of glute strength and we'll reinforce that importance here. If the glutes are strong and equal then the other main muscles of the legs are able to work effectively and efficiently. For most people the glutes are weaker on one side and this has a ripple down effect on the rest of the muscles. What often happens is that the piriformis, IT band and outside hamstring muscle will shorten and tighten up which outwardly rotates the upper leg. Accordingly, the inside of the calf will then tighten up in an attempt to get you realigned by inwardly rotating the lower leg (this is what usually leads to issues such as overpronation, Achilles pain and ankle issues, all of which we'll cover in the next chapter). This inward rotation of the lower leg in reaction to the outward rotation of the upper leg is the body doing its best to get you realigned but it takes the knee joint out of its optimal position when the foot strikes the ground and places it under more stress than is ideal. As a sidenote the same issues would also be occurring when you're walking but as the forces at play in walking are usually much lower, nearer two times your body weight rather than seven times, it may go unnoticed completely or discomfort may only be felt when walking on difficult terrain or up and down steps or hills.

So, where does this battle of inward and outward rotation leave the knee joint? It often results in the knee dropping inwards slightly when the foot strikes the ground. This in itself can overstretch the inside of the knee so some clients will present with pain in that area. For most though the discomfort is on the outside of the knee joint, below the knee joint or a combination of the two. This is due to inflammation in the area caused by the shorter, tightened IT band pulling against its attachment below the knee and this is 'runner's knee' in action. Yet again we find another example here where *pain is just the symptom* and all the while the cause is keeping quiet and going under the radar. The pain occurs due to the IT band attachment becoming irritated and inflamed so the worst thing you could do is irritate it further. Unfortunately, that's what most people do either by digging around and poking the knee or by squatting down or deeply flexing the knee to 'free it up' (doing a quad stretch by bringing your heel to your bum for example). If an area is irritated you need to work on the cause of the irritation so with this example I'd recommend, carefully and lightly initially, foam rolling the IT band to release the tightness (I'd also treat that area as well as the calves and hamstring). Usually, if you foam roller the IT band on the opposite leg you find that it's fine compared to the tight side so that only reaffirms that there is an underlying imbalance at play. I recommend clients to ice the knee if it's sore but we rarely work directly on the joint as it would likely only irritate it further. The long-term solution would be and usually is for most lower body issues, stronger and equal glutes because then you have the best chance of being neutral and allowing all the muscles of the legs to work equally. A brief period of time away from running will often benefit but it doesn't mean all activities have to stop as swimming and cycling, for example, are often still fine to do.

One last point to mention is footwear. We'll talk about it more in the next chapter but if you are experiencing pain because of misalignment then buying new trainers isn't going to balance you up. At best the new sole may provide some extra cushioning but in reality it's much more important that you sort your alignment out and then get new shoes once you are neutral. I've lost count of the times I've heard, "I bought some new trainers a couple of weeks ago because I had my other ones for years and thought they might be the problem but it hasn't made any difference." I don't blame people for trying it but it never works because mechanically you haven't made any significant changes and, as such, your body won't be in a better physical position for having new shoes.

Tips:

- Walk as a warm-up for running – don't just go straight into running.
- Don't just go for a 5K run out of nowhere. Try and gradually build up your distance. The fact you could run 10K a year ago doesn't matter if you haven't run for an entire year since.
- Try and mix up the surfaces that you run on i.e. don't always run on the pavement.
- Don't stretch the quads when running (more on that later).
- Don't go digging around and poking the knee if it's sore.
- Don't buy new shoes unless you're sure your body is in a neutral place.

Some exercises/sports (including those where you're predominantly right or left-footed)

If we were to go through the stresses on the knee in every sport we'd be here forever. We just covered running and I suggested cycling as a good option. I stand by that but I have had a few clients with knee discomfort over the years from cycling (myself included) due to an incorrect saddle height. If the saddle is too low then you can flex your knees too much and then the repeated action of that over thousands of revolutions can eventually create stress around the joint, so if you're unsure get yourself fitted at a bike shop. I also suggested swimming and again I stand by that but I have also had clients where swimming has caused knee discomfort. This has always been due to breaststroke and is another example of an action exaggerating an underlying issue. We said earlier that if the glutes aren't strong enough then the piriformis and IT band will shorten and outwardly rotate the upper leg and so when you think about the breaststroke movement in terms of the upper leg you can see how this would be accidentally reinforcing the tightness in the piriformis and IT band as you actively outwardly rotate the upper leg as part of the movement. A simple fix is just sticking to straight legs when swimming (when doing my rehab I used to do a hybrid stroke of moving my arms as if I were doing breaststroke and my legs as if doing front crawl) because then the knee is tracking neutrally again.

With some sports the stress on the knee is clear to see. We've already mentioned the triple jump as an example and, likewise, it doesn't take much to visualise the stress on a fast bowler's knee in cricket when they plant their front foot to deliver the ball. Some actions in sport are what they are and all you can do is manage the body as best you can and ensure everything is working as equally and efficiently as possible around the sport. Football is another hard one because most players do tend to have a dominant leg and will pass and shoot more with that leg. With football, as well as with other sports that involve kicking actions, the quads can eventually shorten and tighten up so much that they pull against the patella tendon (patella tendonitis). Here, inflammation and pain are felt below the kneecap in the tendon. Nowadays, the best approach to solve this is to foam roll the quads to gradually loosen them so they stop pulling against the tendon. With proper management through stretching, strengthening and foam rolling this issue can be resolved over time.

Moving away from sports, people often experience knee pain when doing activities such as lunges or squats. Although, in theory, these are exercises that should strengthen your glutes the reality is that sometimes people simply aren't strong enough to do them and doing the exercise unintentionally highlights that. We've already said how the IT band likes to take over if the glutes aren't strong enough and it's often the IT band pulling against the knee (like we saw with 'runner's knee') that causes the discomfort when lunging and squatting. With squats, like standing, your weight should be distributed equally 50/50 on both legs. However, if you are slightly out of balance, say 53/47, then your squatting technique will reflect that. Expanding on this example further if your left glute were weaker then you'd squat down slightly more to the left-hand side and your left IT band would have to work harder to keep you in line. The chances are that you wouldn't know you were squatting incorrectly until the knee pain was felt but it's a massive indicator that you're out of balance. As a side note, if both knees hurt when squatting you could be going deeper than your body wants you to go (I don't recommend anyone going any deeper than 90 degrees) or you could be lifting a weight that's too heavy for you. With lunges clients will always say they're more wobbly on the side that the knee hurts. So, say you had a weaker left glute again, when you lunge forward with the left leg you'd be more wobbly because the glute wouldn't stabilise the hip enough, the IT band would have to take over and you'd feel the knee pain as it pulls against the attachment. As long as I feel it's safe for them to do so (i.e. they don't have a potential or underlying issue with the joint) I nearly always get new clients to do a few single leg squats on each leg as this tells me a lot about how things are firing. Most people are more wobbly on one side and struggle to keep the knee pointing forwards through the whole movement. You don't need to do a deep single leg squat to get an idea of what's firing. Most clients just think their balance is bad but when you connect all the dots 99% of the time it all links into the weaker glute on that side. Very occasionally people are equally poor on both sides but at least they are equal so then it's just a case of strengthening rather than realignment first before strengthening. This sense of being wobbly/unstable on one side more than the other can be felt in many more exercises than just lunges but it's an easy one to visualise.

Tips:

- If you're getting knee pain while cycling then check whether you'd benefit from adjusting the saddle height slightly.
- Swimming with straight legs reduces stress on the knees.
- If you're more wobbly on one side than the other then don't just assume it's to do with your balance. It could well be to do with muscular and strength imbalances.

Sleeping

Sleeping tends to be more an issue if you already have knee pain. For example, if you've injured your medial knee ligament you could wake up in agony in the night just because you've been lying with your knees together and the gentle pressure is enough to cause pain. As such, I'd often recommend people with this issue to sleep with a pillow between their knees as a short-term solution to reduce the chances of discomfort. Similarly, sometimes people will struggle to sleep with their knees out straight so if you lie on your back then having a pillow under your knees can help. The only time I think sleeping position can really influence the knee is if you sleep on your front with one knee bent up and out to the side. If you were to stay in that position all night every night then the inside of the knee would have something to say about it in the end.

Tips:
- See if using a pillow for support helps with discomfort.
- Try altering your sleep position to see if it alleviates discomfort.

Cartilage issues/injuries

Much of the advice surrounding knee surgery mirrors that found in the 'hip replacement' section in the last chapter so, to avoid repetition, we'll summarise here rather than go over the same information.

The same key points are relevant with knee surgery. Without wishing to take any credit away from the surgeon, the success of the operation as a whole is widely determined by the work you do before and after the surgery. In relation to issues with damaged cartilage, trimming away the damaged cartilage will undoubtedly have a positive effect on the joint space and functionality. But if the original issue occurred due to years of unequal wear due to misalignment then if nothing changes with the cause, the symptom may return again years down the line. In contrast, if everything were neutral before and the injury occurred due to trauma of some kind then there wouldn't need to be any significant alignment changes post-surgery. However, the challenges of rebuilding the strength and efficiency around the joint on the injured leg and ensuring that the other leg doesn't take over too much throughout the recovery will always be present. If the operation is required due to a trauma injury then you likely won't get much time before the operation to build up your strength. If it's more of a long-term issue and you've been given a date for the operation a few months in advance then there is an opportunity to ensure everything is the best it can be beforehand rather than simply waiting and counting down the days until the operation. Although pain may well limit some capabilities, there are usually many activities that can still be undertaken, either as normal or with adaptations, that can allow you to maintain strength in the surrounding muscles of the knee.

Where this operation is generally less intrusive and traumatic to the body than other knee surgery, the recovery times are usually much quicker. You are encouraged to weight bear relatively quickly post-surgery so this reduces the potential time spent favouring the other leg.

ACL injuries

Anterior Cruciate Ligament (ACL) injuries are, unfortunately, quite common in sport. Contact sports increase the risk but it isn't unheard of that people suffer the injury simply jumping, landing or twisting, with no one else around them. As we mentioned earlier, sometimes there can be unknown underlying imbalances at play, sometimes it's just bad luck and sometimes it's a combination of the two. The severity of the injury is determined through imaging scans and you can have partial ruptures or full ruptures. Depending on the severity of the partial tear and trauma to the surrounding soft tissue, surgery isn't always necessary. If it is determined that the ACL is intact enough then a rehabilitation programme alone is often the recommended approach to avoid the risks associated with surgery. If it has fully ruptured then surgery, followed by a rehabilitation programme, is the usual plan of action. I've seen numerous clients over the years who have had ruptured ACLs and often there is a long wait between diagnosis and surgery. As long as the exercises are safe and suitable (you wouldn't consider lunges for example) we work on maintaining as much strength as we can in the surrounding muscles prior to the surgery and this can result in quicker than average returns to exercise and sports post-surgery.

We seem to be mentioning luck a lot with knees but it is one of those areas where there are so many different ways that trauma can occur that it can simply come down to the angle that you're hit from, or if and how your foot is planted, that determines the severity of the injury and thus the length of your recovery. If the ACL is the only damaged structure then this allows the quickest recovery. If you've been unlucky enough to suffer damage to the cartilage or one or more of the surrounding ligaments as well then this inevitably adds more months to your recovery.

But sometimes things aren't simply down to luck. I've had a couple of clients and have also read of some athletes who, in later life, have had to have knee procedures and it's become apparent that they've been living with a ruptured ACL for years and not even known. Scans reveal the historical rupture that had gone unnoticed due to the strength and stability that they had maintained around the knee joint. I haven't included this observation to dismiss the importance of the ACL. The reason for mentioning it is to reinforce the argument for the importance of the strength and alignment of the surrounding, stabilising structures of the knee.

Knee replacement surgery

As with hip replacements, knee replacement surgery is evolving all the time. The technological advances mean that recovery times are potentially shorter now than ever before. The biggest hope I have for knee and hip replacement surgery is that we can change the presumption, "it's likely that the other side will need doing one day as well." I look at the success of surgery in terms of how it improves the individual as a whole. So, for me, I'm not sure that having a knee replacement, then leaning on the other leg for a few years until the stress on that knee joint is such that it also requires replacing, would be classed as successful. It may not be quite as simple as that for everyone but in many cases I fear that it could be. If all the attention of the rehabilitation is placed on one area (i.e. the replacement knee joint) then stresses on the opposite leg could well be going unnoticed.

I know that the rehabilitation involved after knee replacement surgery is intense as I have worked through this with a few clients over the years. However, having to do it all over again a few years later on the other side isn't any less intense and I'm not sure it gets any easier second time around. I'm passionate about getting everyone to view the body as a whole so, although it may require a few extra strengthening and stretching exercises through your rehabilitation, focusing on the unoperated leg as much as the operated leg can have huge positive implications for your future.

General Tips

We have to start this section with a reminder for standing and sitting correctly. The more time we spend in a neutral balanced position the better it is for all of our joints. I think a big tip for the knees is to not assume that there's something wrong with the joint straight away. If one knee hurts and not the other, which is most likely the case, then you're probably misaligned so shelling out £100 on some new trainers isn't likely to get you the result you desire. When one knee hurts it's often the body hinting at misalignment but most people get drawn into focusing on the knee as the problem. I wonder how many unnecessary knee scans and injections take place every day due to the focus being placed solely on the joint. If the knee is sore don't try and 'free it up' by stretching the joint or overly flexing the joint (i.e. quad stretches, kicking your heels up or squatting down). If you've got a foam roller check to see if the calves and IT bands feel equal side to side. If everything is equal then you may well have an issue with the joint but the chances are you're just out of balance.

What not to do

We've just mentioned this but don't try and 'free up' the knee joint. Unless you are doing a sport where your quads do shorten up (e.g. football or kickboxing) don't stretch your quads as this will usually only add more stress to the joint. Avoid doing similar actions such as squatting down to flex the knee or kicking your heels up. The *if it hurts don't stretch it* rule definitely applies here. If there is already inflammation due to stress from the dysfunctional surrounding muscles then poking and prodding around only adds to the chances of creating more inflammation.

What to do

Knee stability and alignment always starts at the glutes for me. Of course, quad strength is also essential in both the alignment and stabilisation of the knee but the most common factors inhibiting quad strength are tight hip flexors and tight hamstrings. So, with that in mind, we loop back to glute strength being the key again as the most common cause of hamstring and hip flexor tightness is the pelvic rotation associated with glute strength imbalance and weakness. The IT band tightening is another common consequence so foam rolling the IT band is usually effective in alleviating some knee discomfort. Again, it isn't the long-term solution but if you roller both sides and find that there is a difference side to side then you get the diagnostic benefit of using the roller as well as the physical benefits.

Other factors

You know by now that each chapter aims to cover the most familiar challenges facing each area of the body so there will always be a few issues that don't make the cut and get the full attention. We all have small, fluid-filled sacs called bursae that help to provide cushioning for the joints and the knee joint is no exception. As such, bursitis (inflammation of the bursae) is another knee complaint that can causes discomfort and this is often caused by jobs or activities that require prolonged and/or repetitive kneeling. Management of bursitis often revolves around a change of position or activity to reduce the stress from kneeling. Another significant source of knee discomfort is a dislocated knee cap. Anyone who has suffered this will confirm that it is extremely painful and due to the visual deformity of the knee joint, not difficult to diagnose. It usually occurs due to a trauma while twisting so sports are a more probable cause rather than day to day activities. As horrible an injury as it is, if it is solely a dislocation of the kneecap then often the structure of the knee joint itself isn't affected. However, as with any dislocation, if it happens once the chances of it reoccurring do increase but, as always, you can reduce your chances by ensuring all the surrounding structures are working as efficiently as possible.

One final knee issue to mention is Osgood-Schlatter's disease where pain is felt at the attachment of the patellar tendon to top of the tibia (shinbone). For the those with the condition it's usually aggravated by higher impact and activity levels. It's most commonly found in children going through growth spurts and, as such, pain usually subsides once the growth spurts are over. However, in addition to the passing of time, reducing the effect of tight muscles pulling against the area is proven to have a significant impact on reducing symptoms so, like so many other conditions, it's not something to just put up with and wait until it goes away by itself.

Chapter 8

Ankles, Heels and Feet

We started at the top and now we've made it down to the bottom. The ankle joint is incredible when you think about how small it is in relation to what it has to support above it. A lot of the stresses we've covered through the hip and knee sections overlap with the ankle joint as well but there are a couple of issues unique to the ankle and foot. Most of us have felt that sickening feeling of going over on your ankle. Depending on the severity of the roll you've probably seen one of your ankles balloon up and maybe even turn all the colours of the rainbow with bruising. It's incredible how quickly the ankle swells up. Most rugby and football players are familiar with the challenge of trying to take a boot off at the end of a game after an earlier mid-game ankle roll has resulted in the ankle feeling twice the size as normal. More often than not, once the boot is removed, you actually get to see that the ankle really is twice the size due to the swelling. Alas, ankle rolls are not merely confined to sports. Many a client, including myself, has gone over on their ankle by missing a step, going over on uneven ground or even simply just twisting it while walking along on flat, even surfaces. Sometimes it's pure bad luck (e.g. falling down a hole that you didn't know was there) but more often than not it may have been avoidable if the body had been working more efficiently. We'll cover this in greater detail later in this chapter in the *'Regularly Twisting/ Going Over on the Ankle'* section.

Although people have been twisting their ankles since the dawn of time the management and rehabilitation advice has changed in recent times. The acronym RICE (Rest, Ice, Compression, Elevation) goes hand-in-hand with a twisted ankle and, unless in more extreme circumstances where hospitalisation is required, it's a great place to start. Most people are good at this stage but the one area where improvements can often be made is with the elevation. For the elevation to be truly effective I recommend to clients that they need to have their ankle high enough that it's above their heart. Having your ankle resting on the foot stool in front of you isn't high enough for it to be fully effective. You need to be lying on your back with your ankle above your heart so that you get gravity working on your side. I also find that the other temptation at this point is for people to start rotating their ankle around to try and 'free it up' as it feels so stiff. This is another one of those counterintuitive reactions from our brains. If we have just twisted our ankle, possibly tearing a ligament or two in the process and our body has reacted by making the joint massively inflamed to, among other things, avoid any further damage to the joint then overstretching it by rotating it is only likely to damage it further. A part of our brain tries to tell us that we need to free it up, reduce the stiffness and get it moving again but, certainly in the initial stages, that just isn't the case.

The next biggest change to rehabilitation is the timeframe in which you want to start putting more weight through the joint again (i.e. the *rest* phase). For many it's a lot sooner than you may think. The days of putting your feet up for a week to let it heal are long gone. This is a bit of a generalisation and please don't make this decision without getting advice beforehand but in many cases you want to be trying to lightly put weight through the ankle again after around 48 hours if not sooner. The earlier you start using it again the sooner you can start to build your strength and confidence and the quicker you'll recover. Although there are numerous factors at play when rehabilitating an ankle issue I find that one of the biggest blocks to a timely recovery is waiting too long initially to start the rehabilitation. I still hear of people being advised to keep their weight off the ankle for at least a week and that is very, very rarely the right thing to do. It's more often the case that the longer you leave it before starting to challenge the ankle again the longer your recovery will take.

I'm not sure if this point is a change to advice or more of a realisation of the importance of it in recent times but restrengthening the ankle joint after an injury is massively important. Unfortunately, I've seen many clients where this hadn't been emphasised to them in the past and, as such, they have come to see me because they've either reinjured the same ankle again or, maybe even more likely, they've injured something on the opposite leg as they've accidentally been favouring the other side for months when the original ankle injury still hasn't been sorted. I've had many clients who have presented with sciatic nerve irritation or back pain on one side and it turns out the key is an ankle injury from months or even years earlier on the other side. Another common presentation is clients turning up after they've rolled their ankle for the second time. They'll often tell me that they thought it was fixed as it happened a couple of months ago (maybe even longer for some) but it transpires that they hadn't done any strengthening after the original injury and had determined it was fixed because the swelling had gone away and it looked normal again.

When it comes to strengthening it needs to be specific to the injury you've got so I can't cover all eventualities here but I'll explain more in the *'Regularly Twisting/Going Over on the Ankle'* section later on. One point that needs reemphasising though is rotating the ankle to try and get range of movement back isn't an effective part of rehab. I want you to imagine the ligaments like a bit of Blu Tack that has been overstretched, damaged and possibly torn completely due to the trauma of twisting the ankle. If you then twist or rotate your ankle to loosen it up then all you end up doing is recreating the same stress on the ligaments. If you broke your hand by punching a brick wall you wouldn't go back and punch the wall again a few days later to try and make it feel better. The hard bit is that you may find yourself doing it without even really noticing so it's really important to focus on not overstretching the ankle even further when it's already damaged.

So far, the introduction has been a little ankle-heavy so let's talk about the heel a bit and, more specifically, the Achilles tendon. If I could pick a textbook example of *'if it hurts don't stretch it'* in action then Achilles tendon pain would be number one on the list. I am forever having to stop people from stretching out their sore Achilles. I am aware that it is a physical possibility for the Achilles tendon to be short and tight (a 100m sprinter springs to mind as someone where this could be a possibility). However, in over a decade, I have yet to tell a client to stretch their Achilles. I'm sure it will happen one day, probably after I've finished writing this chapter but, to date, I have never seen a client with a short Achilles tendon. I have, however, seen many clients with an overstretched, inflamed Achilles tendon. We'll go into more detail in the 'Achilles tendonitis' section later but it's usually the case that the Achilles is sore, inflamed and overstretched due to a short and tight calf muscle. As such, further stretching out of the already overstretched tendon often does more harm than good or, in a best-case scenario, it's the equivalent of two steps forward and one and three-quarters back. You need to be able to alter the state of the calf without adding further stress to the Achilles and that's where a combination of hands-on treatment and using the foam roller comes in to its own.

Let's look at feet now. I'm not a podiatrist so I don't see a massive variety of feet issues. The most common challenge I face is the effects and complications surrounding low arches or flat feet. It must be said that I have seen a couple of clients over the years where high arches have been a problem but I have seen countless more with issues linked to low arches. Of these clients there have been a couple who have had collapsed arches so I work with them, alongside a podiatrist, to ensure that we can manage the effects and challenges associated with this to ensure as little impact as possible. In contrast, it's been the case that for the vast majority of those (myself included) who I've seen with low arches, flat feet and feet pain these issues are just their symptom. For these people by making everything else in the network more efficient, we've been able to get them out of pain and, for most, allowed them to no longer need supportive insoles and get back into neutral footwear.

The reason I refer to the pains as the symptoms rather than the cause is that most people have lower arches/flat feet due to overpronating. We touched on this a little in the last chapter but most people will be overpronating (by inwardly rotating the lower leg) as a consequence of an externally rotated upper leg. This external rotation in itself is usually a consequence of poor glute functionality on the affected side. Once again, you can see how interconnected the network is so that's why, in my opinion, you have to work on maximising your own efficiency and functionality before looking to external aids to sort you out. Will spending £200 on insoles make your glutes work or is it worth trying to make them stronger first to see if you can get yourself aligned? Also, I can't remember ever seeing a client where both Achilles tendons were equally inflamed or where both arches are equally as painful. That in itself is a massive clue that there is an imbalance so is it worth spending £150 on trainers that offer massive arch support for overpronation when the chances are only one foot needs the support? Do you then accidentally weaken the more efficient side by letting it become reliant on the arch support? What happens when you want to wear flip-flops or walk around barefoot and don't get any support? I'm aware this can sound a little like 'you can strengthen your way out of any issue' and I know that isn't always the case. But I truly believe that we can all make improvements and believe strongly in looking at the network as a whole rather than throwing time and money solely at the symptom. If you can become more efficient further up the network then you can hopefully eventually get to a place of neutral foot strike. This in itself promotes even more efficiency in the network as a whole. More importantly, it also greatly reduces your risk of ankle, heel and feet pain as your body weight is spread more efficiently across your feet and you reduce the risk of twisting your ankle as your foot is landing neutrally on the floor.

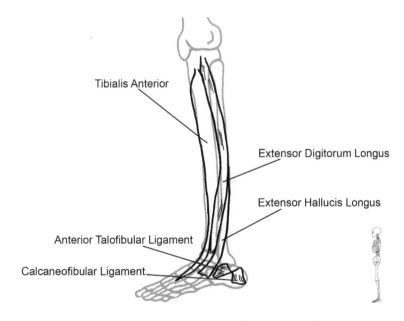

Image 11 – anterior lower leg and ankle

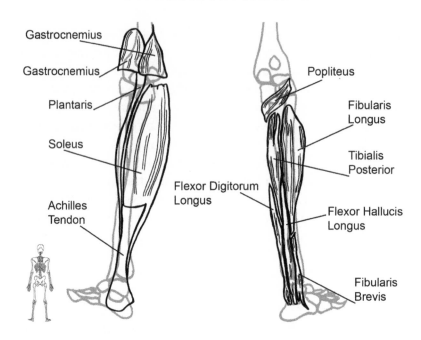

Gastrocnemius
Gastrocnemius
Plantaris
Soleus
Achilles Tendon
Popliteus
Fibularis Longus
Tibialis Posterior
Flexor Digitorum Longus
Flexor Hallucis Longus
Fibularis Brevis

Image 12 – posterior lower leg and ankle

Common Challenges

The biggest challenges to the ankles, heels and feet come from the stresses and inefficiencies further up the network that then result in stress in these areas. It's not really so much of an anterior versus posterior challenge as per some other areas of the body. It's more about how neutrally the foot strikes the ground unconsciously (due to the efficiency of the network as a whole) combined with how neutrally we can keep the ankle and foot when doing activities consciously. So below are the most common areas in which I see ankle, heel and foot pain with clients. As with the chapters beforehand I can't include every single cause of pain I've ever seen so I've picked those that I've seen most frequently:

• standing incorrectly (including gardening, DIY and household chores)
• sitting incorrectly (sofa, desk/work setup etc.)
• driving

- running
- some exercises/sports (especially those where you're predominantly right or left-footed).

Standing incorrectly (including gardening, DIY and household chores)

It really would be a case of repeating myself if I did a massive section here because we really have covered the importance of this in the previous two chapters. However, I make no apologies for mentioning it again briefly here because it is so important. There are rare occasions when we do need to lean on one leg more than the other (taking more weight through one leg to protect the other injured leg for example). Those rare exceptions aside, standing up equally is the way to go. You'll find that as you get better with it that eventually it will feel really weird to lean on one hip. Although you might have had a really long, tiring day gardening or doing some DIY, when you catch yourself doing a cheeky lean in the evening hopefully it would feel strange and uncomfortable because you've trained yourself to be neutral. We've said that no single exercise or stretch is more important than anything else but hopefully you've got the message by now that standing up equally is massive.

Tip:
- You know the drill – tense those glutes and stand up straight!

Sitting incorrectly (sofa, desk/work setup etc.)

Like we said in the last section on standing correctly, we have covered sitting incorrectly in quite some detail over the past two chapters but it's worth reminding ourselves of its importance. Also, it's worth reminding ourselves that we are not robots and we can't be expected to be in the 'perfect' position at all times. I've lost count the amount of times I've uncrossed my ankles while writing this book. Is there a 'perfect' position anyway? If we're feeling a bit ill, for example, do we really want to be sat up perfectly straight on the sofa or do we want to snuggle in instead and feel a bit sorry for ourselves? The idea is to try and ensure we're in the best position we can be in for our body for as much of the time as possible but, inevitably, it isn't feasible or realistic for that to be all day every day. However, if you have an ankle issue and you're accidentally reinforcing the cause of the issue by sitting with your ankles crossed over each other, then making a slight change could have a massive impact. If your office chair encourages you to tuck or cross your ankles then a different chair could be the answer. If you always sit on the same spot on the sofa, then changing where you sit or breaking up your sitting by lying on the floor could stop you from keeping your ankles in a fixed, incorrect position for extended periods of time. Don't beat yourself up if you keep catching yourself returning to the incorrect position either because doing something about it is the key here. I'm making up numbers here but, hypothetically, if you go from crossing your ankles 100 times per day down to 50 times per day that's a massive improvement not just to the amount of times you do it but also to the length of time you spend doing it. If you're consciously aware of it then you're more likely to catch yourself doing it sooner and make the change quicker rather than noticing after half an hour when your ankle aches. It's all about trying to be aware of your body position as often as you can and trying to reduce potentially unnecessary, avoidable stress on our bodies.

Tips:

- Try to mix up where you sit on the sofa to make sure you're not always sat at the same angle.
- Try to try to not cross your feet or legs when you are sat and try to sit equally on each glute.
- Make sure you take regular breaks if you're doing activities that require kneeling or squatting for lengthy periods.

Driving

We have covered a lot of the potential challenges of driving in the last two chapters (including seat position, hitching the hip up and seat height) but there are a couple of foot-specific challenges that are worth a mention. The first of these is the position of the foot on the pedal. You might assume that you push equally with your foot through the pedals but it's worth checking because it isn't always the case. If you have a previous injury that affects how much pressure you can put through certain areas of the foot then of course adjustments have to be made as safety is important. But even if there isn't a reason for you to adjust your foot position it's not guaranteed that you spread your weight evenly through the inside and outside of the foot and you might be surprised to see how your foot makes contact with the pedal. If you have slightly short calves, for example, you might find that you push a lot more through your toes and that there isn't much of your foot actually in contact with the pedal. Likewise, many clients report that they drive more on the inside of their foot with their big toe taking most of the pressure while others may drive with more pressure going through the outside of the foot. As we touched on earlier, safety is important so don't try and make any drastic changes but it could be that the forces you apply through your foot are accidentally reinforcing underlying imbalances.

A different challenge is faced by those driving automatic cars primarily but also those who do lots of motorway driving. If it's a right-hand drive car some people find that they tuck their left foot out the way when it's not being used. Although there isn't much physical stress on the ankle by doing this, as no weight is being put through the joint, it does mean that much like crossing your ankles when sat, you can end up spending prolonged periods of time with the ankle fixed in a poor position. This can be easily rectified by ensuring that the left foot is kept in a neutral position even when not being used.

Tips:

- Check whether your foot position on the pedal could be the cause of, or a contributor towards, any underlying issues.
- Try to keep both feet in a neutral position even if you are only using one for driving.

Running

We said in the last chapter that knee issues are the most familiar challenges faced by runners. I would say that ankle, heel and foot issues aren't that far behind on the list though. Due to dysfunction elsewhere in the network one foot taking more bodyweight over the other, alongside one or both feet not striking the ground neutrally, forms a perfect recipe for discomfort at the ankles, heels and feet. We'll cover each of the issues individually later in the chapter but the most common symptoms that occur due to this are Achilles' tendonitis, plantar fasciitis, twisted ankles and shin splints. Each of these come from the similar cause of misalignment in the network filtering down to the feet. This misalignment is then compounded further by the relentless incorrect foot striking that occurs though running, in combination with the increased stress put through the area in running (around seven times your bodyweight). It's this combination of factors that lead to so many areas of the lower leg being put under stress hence the variety of issues that can occur.

Although efficient functionality will always be the dominating factor in reducing the risk of injury, there are a couple of other foot specific factors we can consider. Firstly, the terrain on which you're running can have varying levels of significance. For example, if you have an overstretched Achilles tendon then running up hills could irritate this further as the angle of the foot strike would be stretching the tendon even more. Another factor that can affect foot strike is if you always run on the same side of the road or, which is more likely to be the case, you run the same routes that mean you're on one side of the road more than the other. This means that the camber of the pavement and the impact of the dropped kerbs will affect one side more than the other if you always follow the same route. Fortunately, if you're partial to following the same route then there is a simple solution – run the route the other way. The surface that you're running on can also make a difference. If an area is already inflamed, such as the plantar fascia with plantar fasciitis, then running on firm, unforgiving surfaces could add more irritation compared to running on softer, more forgiving surfaces. Conversely, if you have an ankle issue due to overpronating and are susceptible to rolling your ankle then you may find trail running too difficult and may prefer running on a smooth, consistent surface. As with most situations these factors only play a part because the body isn't working efficiently in the first place and they are rarely the main cause of an issue in their own right.

Footwear has already been mentioned earlier in the chapter but it's worth revisiting. New shoes are rarely the miracle cure because they don't often have the power to significantly change your functionality. Unfortunately, the only time I've seen footwear have a significant impact on functionality has been the detrimental effects of clients trying barefoot running. It's important to note here that I have never tried this myself so I am basing this on my opinion of the logic behind it and the effects I have seen when clients have tried it. Only a handful have given it a go and it has led to increased stress on their calf muscles where they have lost the cushioning support of normal running shoes and their calves have had to work much harder. The increased stress was also felt equally so it confirms that the shoes were the cause as opposed to underlying imbalances. It could be coincidence of course that the same issue happened because it wasn't a massive sample size. However, I've seen enough with those clients who did try it that when clients ask if I would recommend barefoot running I advise them to try and make improvements in their own functionality rather than hoping that shoes will make the difference.

Tips:

- Walk as a warm-up for running – don't just go straight into running.
- Don't just go for a 5K run out of nowhere. Try and gradually build up your distance. The fact you could run 10K a year ago doesn't matter if you haven't run for an entire year since.
- Try and mix up the surfaces that you run on i.e. don't always run on the pavement.
- Don't stretch the Achilles if it's sore (more on that later).
- Don't try to change your foot strike or stride length. It is what it is due to how your body is functioning so if you make improvements in functionality then this will filter down to an improved foot strike and stride length.
- Don't buy new shoes unless you're sure your body is in a neutral place.

Some exercises/sports (especially those where you're predominantly right or left-footed)

Any sport where you have a dominant foot for taking off from, landing on or for kicking with has the potential to put more stress through one foot over the other. With the more obvious examples like high jump, football and kickboxing it's clear that more stress would go through one leg over the other so the risks of injury and overuse are likely to be higher on that side. Sports or activities that require short, sharp movements and quick changes of direction such as netball, tennis and badminton also ask a lot of questions of the lower leg. Combine all those factors with physical contact from opposing players and it's easy to see how feet and ankle issues occur regularly in sports such as football, rugby and netball. Additionally, if you are doing these activities with underlying imbalances these can get accidentally further reinforced simply by playing. For example, if you were a defender in netball and had a tight calf and overstretched Achilles, regularly going up onto your toes to block a shot wouldn't help the situation.

That being said it isn't only sports that can accidentally reinforce problems. If you were prone to overstretching your ankle due to a tight medial (inside) calf then doing a seemingly simple activity like a lunge could be reinforcing those underlying issues and potentially be increasing your risk of injury. If you had a sore, overstretched Achilles then doing dynamic exercises or high-intensity interval training (HIIT) workouts could be inadvertently shortening the calf even more and adding even more stress to the tendon. Similarly, doing weighted versions of activities can help to build muscle mass and tone but if you're misaligned then you might be adding more mass and tone to calf muscle that is already too strong and working too hard. Likewise, if you're squatting from a misaligned position then you could accidentally be putting further stress on the weaker side and therefore increasing the stress on the calf, ankle, foot and heel even though you're trying to do an activity to strengthen the glutes.

These are just a few examples of activities that can inadvertently do more harm than good if done from an incorrect starting position. I'm always saying to clients that it doesn't mean that these are bad exercises – far from it in fact. However, the key factors are whether you're aligned, functional and strong enough for the exercises/sports to be beneficial for you. That's the part that the body won't tell you until often it's too late. You may not know that you overpronate until you try to change direction quickly in netball and go over on your ankle. You may not know that your calf is short and the Achilles tendon overstretched until you feel Achilles pain on one side the day after a HIIT workout. You may not know that the inside of your calf is tight and the plantar fascia overstretched when you're running until the morning after when you try to get out of bed and the sole of your foot feels like it's on fire for the first few steps. The advice is always the same – if in doubt seek professional advice first before finding out the hard way and getting injured.

Tips:

- If you're getting Achilles pain while exercising don't stretch it – there's a good chance that it's overstretched and stretching would make it worse.
- If you seem more unbalanced on one side don't just assume it's do with your sense of balance. It could well be to do with muscular and strength imbalances.

Achilles' tendonitis

As I said earlier in the chapter this is a classic example of *'if it hurts don't stretch it'*. Achilles' tendonitis usually occurs due to months (more likely years) of inefficiencies in the network which lead to the gradual shortening and tightening of the calf and, as a result, the gradual stretching, lengthening and inflammation of the Achilles' tendon. I've never seen a client present with both Achilles' tendons being inflamed equally so this reinforces the main cause being the imbalance and inefficiency of the body as a whole. Of the clients I've seen that present with this issue there has usually been a previous injury on the opposite leg (e.g. an injured ankle, knee or hip from months or years ago) causing them to have favoured the opposite leg until it resulted in the inflamed tendon. There is rarely an exact cause of the tendonitis, such as a specific incident that the client can put their finger on, because it's often due to repeated stress over time. It's the snowball effect in action – the stress and inefficiency gradually builds and builds until a tipping point is reached and pain is felt. It often starts as more of an annoying niggle rather than significant pain. People often find they start to feel it towards the end of a run, after a long day on their feet or notice that it feels stiff first thing in the morning and takes a few steps to get going and feel like they can walk properly. At this point it isn't too disruptive but as it continues getting metaphorically poked with a stick, it becomes increasingly inflamed to a point where it starts to feel sore halfway through a run, or by mid-afternoon on a normal day or it takes a good minute or so in the morning before you can walk freely. Eventually, without intervention, it can lead to continual pain all through the day and activities such as walking or running become intolerable due to the pain.

As with most issues in the body the earlier you start to address it the sooner it can get sorted. The main issue here, much like with rotator cuff tendonitis in the shoulder, is that because there isn't a specific injury as such, or a specific time when the tendon was traumatised most people tend to let it go on for longer than they should in the hope that it'll 'sort itself out'. Suddenly, six months can pass you by in a blink and you're left wishing you'd got it looked at sooner. Another common issue is that rest can trick you in to thinking it's ok. If you start to notice it in the initial stages of irritation when running and then have a week off running then it'll probably feel a bit better. That is until you try and run again and then you can still feel it. In this instance all that rest has achieved is to temporarily stop the Achilles being 'poked with a stick' and nothing has been done to address the actual cause of the inefficiency that has led to the pain.

The next option is usually an internet search for recommendations for dealing with Achilles' tendon pain or seeking advice privately. Here you'll often be met with all sorts of ways to treat the symptoms such as RICE, steroid injections, heel lifts, calf stretching and Achilles strengthening. Very rarely is there advice on addressing the cause. Also, in my opinion, a lot of the advice is counterproductive and can often make your symptoms worse. If we refresh our memories we remember that the main cause of Achilles' tendon pain comes from a short, tight calf pulling against the tendon. Therefore, I'm not sure that a heel lift will help as, although it may temporarily take some of the stress off the tendon, this will only actually lead to further shortening of the calf. Next, stretching out the Achilles is a huge no no. If it is already overstretched and inflamed then how can stretching it further possibly help? I've had so many clients over the years who have been advised by other professionals to stretch their calves and Achilles and most are advised to do it dropping off a step or stair so that they can stretch the Achilles even further! It's infuriating as all it does is irritate their tendon even more. Usually, they are also advised to stretch both sides the same as well which makes even less sense as only one side has the issue. The next equally annoying recommendation is Achilles' strengthening. Firstly, the tendon is inflamed and irritated so why would you want to challenge it further and irritate it more? Secondly, Achilles' strengthening will always involve shortening of the calf muscles – they don't need any reason to become even shorter than they already are. Hopefully the popular advice will change one day and my rants to clients and in this book will be worth it but, currently, most people are generally advised on completely the wrong ways to deal with Achilles' pain. The short-term key is to stop the calf pulling against the Achilles and the best approach to this is a combination of hands-on treatment to the calf and use of the foam roller on the calf to try and loosen it up. If I'm treating someone with Achilles' tendonitis I will possibly do a couple of minutes of treatment on the tendon itself depending on the severity of the inflammation but the majority of the time in the initial sessions is spent working on the calf (the immediate cause). As the symptoms reduce you can then work on what I call the 'bigger picture stuff', so we'd move on to the glute strengthening (the overall cause) and reducing the tightness in the hamstrings and piriformis on that side.

Throughout this book I emphasise the importance of seeking support and advice from a professional. However, if you or someone you know are struggling with this issue and don't seem to be making progress and you/they are being told to stretch the calf and strengthen the Achilles, then it might be worth looking elsewhere for advice.

Plantar fasciitis

Plantar fasciitis is the inflammation of the plantar fascia area between your heel and toes. Pain can be experienced at various points in this area, so its diagnosis can cover a broad area of the foot. Pain is often at its worst first thing in the morning with clients often describing the pain as sharp and feeling as if the bottom of their foot is burning. Once again, this a common issue that I've seen many, many times over the years. Additionally, this is another issue where I have yet to ever see anyone with equal pain in both feet and is another example of an issue caused by underlying imbalances elsewhere in the network. Due to the discomfort being down to dysfunction, the commonly suggested approach of rest, ice and anti-inflammatories doesn't get to the cause of the issue. Much like the case with Achilles' tendonitis, the plantar fascia area is usually put under excess stress due to a combination of factors leading to the shortening of the medial calf and then excess overpronation. To flip it round the other way I never have seen and don't ever expect to see, anyone who is functioning pretty neutrally and efficiently that has plantar fasciitis. Accordingly, by improving the client's efficiency I believe that you can resolve the symptoms and, maybe more importantly, ensure that they don't return.

There are additional factors to consider with plantar fasciitis other than just being as efficient and neutral as you can but I would strongly argue that this is by far the most important factor. Footwear can be something to consider but this is usually only a factor if there has been a sudden change in footwear. For example, if you are used to wearing trainers with lots of arch support and then suddenly change to trainers with little to none, then this could increase the stress on the plantar fascia area. However, if this were the sole cause of the problem then a change of shoes would affect both feet equally and should create equal discomfort on both sides. However, it could potentially exaggerate the underlying imbalance and become a tipping point which is why I think it's worth a mention. Another factor could be a sudden change in work circumstances such as changing from a sedentary job to a job where you're on your feet all day. As with the point on trainers if this were the sole cause of the issue then pain would be felt exactly the same on both feet and this is very rarely the case. Following along the same thread a significant increase in activity levels could be a contributing factor whether that's taking on new activities, significantly increasing existing activity levels or a combination of the two. This would again highlight the underlying imbalances rather than being the sole cause of discomfort.

So, like many other issues already discussed, the key is to improve alignment and efficiency so that any stress on the plantar fascia area leading to the inflammation is reduced. I want to finish this section discussing one bit of common advice that, I feel, is extremely detrimental to progress. We said previously that stretching the already overstretched and inflamed Achilles' tendon further makes things worse but that it is often recommended. I have no idea how this became popular but a suggestion often made for plantar fasciitis is rolling a golf ball under your foot to 'ease the symptoms'. This suggestion doesn't make sense to me. The area must already be in an inflamed and irritated state for pain to be experienced. Rolling a rock-hard golf ball over an already inflamed and irritated area seems ridiculous to me. It seems to me like it's the equivalent of trying to cure a headache by headbutting a wall. The area is already irritated, so I'm not sure how exposing it to even more stress helps. When I'm working with clients with plantar fasciitis (similarly to those with Achilles' tendonitis) depending on the severity of the issue I'll either work on it lightly or I'll leave it alone completely because I don't want to add further stress to the area. Working on the inside of the calf is the key initially before working on the network inefficiencies as a whole. Nowhere in that process is there anything involving battering your foot with a golf ball!

Regularly twisting/going over on the ankle

Our ankles are capable of an extraordinary range of movement when you consider the fact that they have to carry the weight of the body. This can be both a blessing and a curse because although the ankles allow us to be able to adapt to walking on all sorts of different terrains and allow us to move at all kinds of funny angles, they are susceptible to being taken to their extremes more than other joints, especially if they have been injured before. You often hear the phrase 'glass ankles' being thrown around for people who suffer from regular ankle twists and rolls. I myself was part of the 'glass ankle club' when I was a teenager playing football. Me and a couple of fellow members of the club could be walking along the perfectly flat corridor at school and any one of us could just twist our ankles, seemingly out of nowhere. During that time I couldn't understand why I was so unlucky to have such weak joints and I've had similar conversations with other clients regarding their relentless ankle injuries. On a couple of occasions I probably was unlucky (falling down a little hole on the football pitch mid sprint or blocking a clearance in football and tearing the medial ankle ligaments) but I can look back now and understand that most of it wasn't down to bad luck but down to poor strength and alignment. Many people who suffer from recurrent ankle injuries don't do enough ankle-specific strengthening. Like we touched on earlier, strengthening always needs to be specific to the injury you've sustained. Some activities such as a single leg balance or, later on down the line, using a wobble cushion or board are quite generically positive exercises for ankles. However, if you've gone over on your ankle and overstretched the outside of the joint, for example, then you'd do different strengthening (eversion strengthening) compared to if you'd overstretched the inside of the ankle (inversion strengthening) so it's important to be specific with what you do.

As we've covered significantly in this chapter, most lower body issues are down to inefficiencies in the network as a whole so quite often the long-term solution to stopping twisting your ankles isn't ankle strengthening alone but to also making sure you have stronger glutes and, as a result, improved efficiency in the legs leading to a neutral foot strike. If the inside of your calf is tight and you overpronate every step you take then you're increasing your risk of going over on your ankle. In contrast, if your foot strikes the ground neutrally every step then this risk is greatly reduced. Also, striking neutrally reduces the stress on your feet and ankles as a whole. Therefore, if they are working optimally and you do come across something unexpected (e.g. some random uneven ground or slipping off a kerb) you are more likely to be able to get away from that unscathed compared to if you already have tired, weak and chronically overstretched ankle ligaments.

Shin splints

Shin splints aren't really to do with the ankle, heel or foot but they have come up quite a few times over the years so I think it's worth a mention. The most common symptom of shin splints is pain along the medial border of the tibia (the inside of the shin). It's an issue usually caused by repetitive overuse so rest, ice and anti-inflammatories are often advised to treat the symptom. As always there must be a cause for the symptom so just managing pain and resting isn't going to stop it coming back again in the future. In reality I often see that rest doesn't make a massive difference because the underlying issue isn't addressed. Clients will often say they've tried resting for two or three weeks but when they return to activity the discomfort levels are still about the same. I've seen many clients with this issue and much like everything else we've discussed in this chapter I've never had a client where both shins are equally inflamed and irritated. For most clients it's just one shin that is affected. Occasionally clients will have both but with one significantly more uncomfortable than the other. Once again the imbalance in pain levels is a clue to an imbalance in the network as a whole. Without wishing to make it sound like all lower leg issues originate from the same cause, it's most common to have the discomfort due to the medial plantar flexor muscles (inside of the calf) being short and tight and pulling away against the border of the medial tibia. It's this relentless pulling and overstretching that causes the inflammation leading to the pain. The discomfort presents itself in many different forms. Some people describe it as a niggling pain; some as sharp, stabbing pains and others as a continual ache but the remedy is usually the same. If you can stop the medial calf from being short, overworked and pulling against the border of the tibia then you can stop the discomfort. Shin splints are the result of a prolonged period of misalignment so progress, as with most issues, will never be instant. However, through addressing the underlying imbalances, it's realistic to expect to eventually be pain-free and, by addressing the underlying issues rather than simply managing the symptom, you greatly reduce the chances of the issue ever returning again.

General tips

As always, we have to start with trying to stand and sit straight, equally and neutrally as often as you can. The more time you can spend nearer a neutral position the better. With that in mind one side hurting more than the other is often a clue that you're out of alignment.

Sometimes activities and exercises can be contributors but it's rare that they are the only causes.

It's easy to think, "I'm right-footed and I know it's my stronger side so my right calf is bound to be tighter" or "My right leg was my stronger leg when I used to play sports so my left ankle probably just hurts when I run because it's my weaker side." That second thought in particular catches a lot of people out. Sure, you may feel comfortable kicking a ball with one foot over the other but that doesn't mean that one leg is, or should be, stronger than the other. On a few occasions in a sporting scenario one side may get used more than the other but the rest of the time you should be aiming for equal strength and functionality. Going back to the first thought, the short calf could be an indicator of a short hamstring on the same leg, a weaker glute on that side and, as such, a clue that you could in fact actually be weaker on that supposed 'stronger side'. Using the foam roller on the calves to see if there is a difference medially and laterally (inside and outside) and any difference between the left and the right can help you to work out if there are bigger imbalances at play.

Just like every other body part we've covered so far it can be easy to obsess over treating the symptom while potentially missing the cause. Rest and ice often make only a minor difference and having a cortisone injection in your ankle, Achilles' tendon or plantar fascia is often only firefighting and unlikely to change the cause of your issue. Where many ankle and foot issues can be chronic in nature it's easy to hope they'll go away by themselves or expect things to change significantly with a couple of weeks rest. This is very rarely the case so if you feel like you're stuck in a cycle of pain with one of these issues then I always think it's best to try and get advice from someone who looks at the whole chain of events rather than someone who just zooms in on the symptom.

What not to do

In short don't focus all your efforts on the symptom alone as in many cases the commonly suggested approaches can do more harm than good. If your Achilles is sore don't stretch it as it's likely that it's already overstretched. If your plantar fascia area is sore then don't batter it with a golf ball as it's already inflamed. If you've gone over on your ankle then don't twist it or roll it further to try and 'free it up' as it's already been overstretched. These are all examples once again of the *'if it hurts don't stretch it'* rule in action. Also, specifically looking at the Achilles' tendon, it's often a bad idea to do Achilles' strengthening exercises as all they tend to do is make the calf shorter and add more stress to the already irritated Achilles' tendon.

The chances are that if you're suffering with one of these issues then only one side hurts, or at least one side hurts significantly more than the other, which confirms that misalignment is a significant factor. With that in mind, spending a lot of money on a pair of insoles or some new trainers isn't going to sort out that misalignment as any changes from either of those would affect both sides equally. I'd always suggest holding off doing anything like that until you've found out if you're working efficiently or not. You will likely find that once your imbalances are addressed and functionality improves, the symptoms will gradually ease and eventually disappear completely.

What to do

The way to successfully address imbalances always involves a combination of specific stretches and strengthening. If it transpires that one glute is weaker than the other side and that is accompanied by a shorter hamstring, piriformis, IT band and medial calf, then targeted stretching, foam rolling and strengthening can hopefully address all the imbalances over time.

If an ankle ligament injury has occurred then strengthening will be required. The strengthening needs to be specific to the injury that has occurred (i.e. medial ligament injuries need slightly different exercises to lateral ligament injuries) especially in the initial stages of rehabilitation. This is different to the Achilles advice because in the ankle scenario the ligament will have been damaged and therefore needs to be restrengthened. With the Achilles tendon, unless it has been torn, strengthening is rarely the correct plan of action.

Other factors

The Achilles' tendon can tear partially or completely so that's why you hear the terms partial rupture or full rupture when referring to this injury. The severity of the injury is determined by a scan and this informs the decision on whether to operate. Most but not all full ruptures result in surgery, whereas partial ruptures may not require surgery at all. The rehabilitation process is a long one and, if surgery has been required, full effectiveness from the surgery is only achieved if it's followed up with a solid effort on the rehabilitation front.

Moving away from the Achilles there are a few other issues that have popped up over the years that are worth a mention. A few clients who primarily run have suffered with a Morton's neuroma. It occurs due to the nerve between two of the toes becoming irritated and they often describe the feeling as if they've got a small stone under their foot. This is usually resolved by a period of rest to reduce the stress on the nerve.

Another issue that usually requires a period of rest is a stress fracture. These are usually caused by repeated overtraining or from a trauma to the foot. Through a reduction in activity intensity the symptoms usually subside within a few weeks but the recovery time is correlated to the severity of the injury.

An issue that can't just be sorted with rest is a bunion – a bony lump that forms on the side of the foot. You can try and make adjustments to manage the issue but in more significant cases surgery is required.

One final issue that has cropped a couple of times with younger clients is Sever's disease. This is where there is a swelling at the growth plate in the heel. This swelling usually occurs due to a combination of high-impact activities being undertaken at the same time as a growth spurt. It's usually managed through a combination of rest, continuing with lower-intensity activities and treating the surrounding areas to ensure there's no further unnecessary excess stress on the growth plate. Recovery time is significantly affected by the length of the growth spurt but it is usually an issue that disappears completely over time.

CHAPTER 9

Frequently Asked Questions

Seeing clients for over a decade means I've been asked all sorts of questions and some do come up more often than others. That's why I thought I'd put this section in at the end.

Some questions are common responses after I explain that it's the overstretched muscles that hurt or when I talk about the importance of standing up straight. Others are just questions that come up regularly and which I think are worth addressing. Let's get started.

"Why does stretching the wrong thing feel so nice?"

This is definitely the most popular question and I understand why. Surely, if it was bad for you and the wrong thing to do, then stretching something that's already overstretched should be agonising and feel like it's making things worse. But instead, unfortunately, it feels lovely and like it's probably doing you some good, so for many it can be a hard habit to break. The biggest problem is that stretching feels nice. If you stretch out in bed before you get up in the morning it feels lovely and you feel better for doing it. For many, though, this could be the first and last stretch they do in a day that is any good for them.

For an area under stress the stress response is often pain. But what the brain doesn't do is connect the dots for you and let you know where the stress is originating from. All you are told is that something is sore and you need to do something about it. You aren't given the full story and because the brain remembers that stretching releases endorphins it guesses that if something is already sore then stretching it more is bound to feel great and it usually does. That's the problem right there. If your lower back is sore (because it's overstretched) and you stretch it out it often feels lovely because you get such an intense stretch. However, all you've actually achieved is to add even more stress by further lengthening an area that is already overstretched. I always ask clients to think about the actual relief that they get by stretching something that's already overstretched, whatever the body part may be. Nearly every time a client will say that they get some instant, temporary relief ranging from just a couple of seconds up to a few minutes but that the pain soon returns. They feel like they get a mini win by stretching but that the issue never really goes away. Most people will also say they feel that the worse the pain is the more they feel they need to stretch it and, as such, they end up stuck in the cycle of stretching the wrong thing by accident even more. That's the key because you're only ever working on the symptom and, usually, making the symptom worse by stretching it. The challenge is to listen to the symptom, take a moment and then try to work out what could be short, assuming that the symptom is already overstretched. If you're used to stretching your neck out when at your desk, for example, it will be tough to break that habit as you're possibly even doing it unconsciously sometimes. But break the habit you must as it will open the door to relieving your pain which leads you on to bigger and better things in the form of strengthening and balance which will then, in turn, greatly reduce the risk of the symptom returning in the future.

"Because I'm leaning on my right leg all the time should I try and lean on the left instead to balance up quicker?"

In a word, no. I think it's a great question though as it shows the client is thinking about how everything works but it's not the way to do it. By leaning on the other leg instead you'd just be swapping the stresses and habits of one side and simply transferring them on to the other side. Think about heating and how you set the thermostat to the temperature that you find comfortable. You wouldn't crank it up really high until it was too hot and then turn it down really low until it was too cold and then keep repeating that process going from one extreme to the other. You find somewhere around the middle that's consistently around the temperature that you find comfortable. We're designed to be neutral so being in a neutral position as often as possible is the key so, when it comes to standing, having 50/50 weight distribution is the goal. We are constantly using our legs independently throughout the day and chopping and changing which side takes more bodyweight. So, when we are stood, if we can give the body some temporary calm by being neutral it makes a dramatic difference.

**"Okay but I'm right-handed and you're saying
I should try and use my left more. Why is that any different?"**

Another great question. When it comes to the upper body most of us do have a more dominant hand and the older we are the longer this dominance will have been present. Throughout the day there aren't many opportunities to do an activity where we use both arms exactly the same with the same amount of strength and muscle activation. The key difference compared to the lower body is that using one side more than the other in the upper body can potentially create a significant difference in strength from one side to the other (whereas in the lower body if you're leaning on one leg then that side is actually the weaker side, so it's more about avoiding stresses and imbalances that can reinforce this weakness). So, when it comes to those rare occasions where we need both sides to work together, if one side is significantly stronger than the other then it will likely take over and further reinforce the imbalance. This could eventually lead to overuse issues in the dominant side or, conversely, when you have to do something where you need both sides to work together (e.g. lifting something heavy that you have to keep level) the weaker, less dominant side may get irritated or even injured. However, if your less dominant side were being asked to work more frequently day-to-day then the risks of either of those issues occurring would reduce significantly as both sides would be closer to equal. It's always worth reminding ourselves that 'closer to equal' is the most likely target with the upper body rather than actually achieving truly equal strength and control with both sides. I'm not saying it's impossible and the younger you are when you start doing this the better. However, if you've been predominantly right-handed for 60 years, for example, then I'm not sure it's realistic to expect to be able to have equal strength in both sides by using your left side more often. Any gains that get you closer to being more balanced and equal shouldn't be laughed at though, so I always encourage everyone to try and make changes, whatever their age. I think it's never too late to start using your less dominant hand so why not step out of your comfort zone and try things like using the remote, brushing your teeth or drinking with your less dominant side. It may feel a bit alien to begin with but, before long, you'll start to feel more confident in the less dominant side and hopefully notice improvements in strength, control and confidence when using that side.

"If you had to pick one what's the most important stretch or strengthening exercise?"

Unfortunately, I think most people that ask this question are doing so from a place of hope that they can get away with just doing one thing per day. I always think fair play for trying but it doesn't work like that I'm afraid! We are complex beings that need to focus on numerous areas all at once. I think it should be a full-time job just to look after ourselves and make sure our bodies are working at their most efficient all the time but alas, for most, that won't pay the bills. I have a loose framework that I work within and, as such, I believe that more strength in certain areas of the body over other areas is key to achieving that longed-for efficiency and strength. From a lower body perspective, glute strength and balance is key. For the upper body, upper back strength and shoulder position are the dominant factors. However, if there was one glute strengthening exercise that guaranteed to keep you strong and neutral forever and one upper back strengthening exercise that ensured perfect shoulder position and balance then we'd all be doing it each and every day and I'd be out of a job. In the same way, contrary to what some adverts will try and tell you, there isn't one superfood that works for everyone or one activity that ensures balanced mental health forever. The reality is that your body and your life are unique so only you face your exact challenges over your lifetime. But the hope is that by reading this book you will become more aware of those challenges you face as an individual and how, potentially, some of the things you're doing that you've been told will help you or that you do out of habit may not actually be having a positive effect on your body. So, in short, I'm afraid that the answer to this question is that there isn't any single activity that's most important. We are incredible machines that require a myriad of processes and functions to be happening all at once so there are lots of areas that all require a bit of our attention. The goal is to avoid one area of the network being under so much stress that it demands all of our attention.

"What glute strengthening exercises should I be doing or avoiding?"

As always the answer to this question has to be based on the individual and their functionality. If someone has relatively good glute functionality then getting them to practice single leg standing to engage the glute may be a little too easy for them. Likewise, if a client is presenting with poor glute functionality and misalignment then an activity such as squats would likely be too difficult for them. First and foremost the main issue with squats in this scenario would be that the individual isn't balanced so, as it's usually a case of the strong get stronger and the weak get weaker with the body then undertaking this exercise would likely increase the underlying imbalance. Combine this with the fact that in all likelihood the glutes wouldn't engage enough in the squat process if they're not strong enough then you could find that the individual can complete the squat movement but to do so they accidentally recruit the wrong muscles as well as doing the action out of balance.

This isn't a criticism of squats as, in the right time and place, they can be a very effective glute strengthening exercise. The key, as with all glute strengthening, is that it really depends on if you're strong enough in the first place for the activity to be beneficial to you. So many times I've seen clients who have been told things like doing lunges will make their knee better but when they try it they find that it makes the issue worse. I've heard countless variations of this in terms of body part and exercise but the reason for the discomfort is usually the same. Even though they're trying to do the right thing in terms of getting stronger and focussing on the glute strengthening the exercise itself is just too difficult for them at that point in time. It's for this reason

I often group glute strengthening exercises into different levels, ranging from easiest to hardest, and make suggestions based on where the individual is starting from. There are so many exercises that engage the glutes that it would be ridiculous to try and include everything but here's an idea of the kind of exercises I talk about most regularly with clients:

- Starting with the more basic and introductory work we're initially just looking at glute activation. This often includes activities such as standing up straight and engaging the glutes, single leg standing with focus on the glute activation and not letting the hip drop and basic hip extension movements to really get used to the feel of the glutes engaging.
- Moving up a step we can then look at introducing some simple movements into the fold so activities such as clams, bridges and 4-point kneeling are often effective here. They require concentration on the glute activation and control throughout so that's why I find these so effective at this stage.
- Once those activities begin to feel easy we can look at slightly more complex movements such as lunges, split squats, single-leg bridges, single-leg deadlifts and single-leg squats. These are a step up from the last level but they are still just body weight exercises and, as many people at this stage may still be slightly out of balance, they can be tailored to a specific ratio as needed as they are all single-leg activities.

After a period of time working on the last group of exercises most clients will eventually get to 50/50 and neutral and from here strengthening can be taken up another level. At this point going up another level can take different forms and the approach that the individual takes often depends on their individual history as well as their end goals. One approach could be to move into activities such as squats and deadlifts and then build up strength through making these weighted. Another approach can be to stay with single-leg work but then find ways to make that more challenging. This could include making the activities weighted to add more resistance or making them more challenging stability wise (by doing them on a wobble cushion or by adding rotation with the upper body for example) or making them more dynamic or explosive (jumping lunges or single leg box jumps for example). You could build up to mixing and matching to make things even more challenging by doing activities such as lunging onto a wobble cushion with a bar bell and then rotating the upper body for example. The variations and adaptations are endless hence this being such a long answer to the original question! I also don't have a preferred method or route of making improvements for clients because it really does depend on the individual situation. If someone is looking to get back to football, for example, then we would most likely tailor their exercises more towards the dynamic and explosive single-leg work but there would still be a place for some double-leg strength work as well.

As we alluded to earlier often the issue can be that an individual is trying to do the right thing in principle but the body just isn't quite strong enough to undertake the activity effectively. That's why it's so important to understand where you're starting from in order to get an idea of what you need to do going forward. If your glutes are weak and you have lower back discomfort on one side then are dead lifts really going to help or could they be reinforcing your issue?

"Should I stretch before exercise?"

This is a tricky one as you could ask 10 health professionals and get 10 slightly different answers so I must stress that this is my opinion here. However, this opinion is based on what I do myself before exercise, as well as what I recommend to all my clients. I know that what I do now is very different to what I used to before I got into this career. Likewise for most clients it is initially a novel approach but it's an approach that I've found to be successful for myself and for them. So again, in short, the answer to "should I stretch before exercise?" is no.

In order to exercise effectively you want the muscles to have a delicate balance of tension and flexibility to have the power and efficiency for the movements required for the specific upcoming exercise. You could imagine the muscles as coiled springs full of potential energy that are ready to allow you to bounce and jump around for your exercise. The muscles need to be warmed up of course (and we'll cover that more with the next question) but if you stretch them out when cold, before you exercise, you're reducing the potential of the spring and forces they can generate. You're essentially stretching out the coiled spring and accidentally reducing the potential spring of the muscles. When I was at school and probably long before I was around, we were told to never bounce when stretching (dynamic stretching) and to always hold your stretches (static stretching) before exercising. At that time those were the best recommendations based on the science available but a lot has changed in the last 20 years. However, although knowledge has improved for some, in terms of the negative effects of static stretching before exercise, the message hasn't reached everyone and many people are still, I feel, stretching incorrectly before exercise. Forcing muscles to lengthen to their maximum when they are cold (i.e. with less blood flow than when exercising) before exercise may increase the chance of injury. You wouldn't intentionally try and pick up something that you knew you was too heavy and impossible for you to lift for fear of getting injured. Yet, for some reason, we expect our muscles to be happy with, out of nowhere, being stretched to their maximum range without any warning. The irony is that doing this only increases your chance of injury and this is just another example of something where, although the intentions may well be positive, the outcomes likely won't be so positive.

"What should I do in my warm-up?"

So, if you're not supposed to stretch before you exercise then what should you do? I think for some, possibly many, a warm-up entails going through the motions of the most common stretches they can remember. It can often be something people feel they should do, rather than something they want to do and, as such, it can be a little brief and relatively ineffective. More importantly, if the warm-up is predominantly made up of static stretches then I would argue that doing nothing would be more beneficial as at least it wouldn't increase your chances of getting injured as much. So now we're back to the original question – what should you do in a warm-up?

The key point and I make no apologies for how obvious this may sound, is that you need to warm-up the muscles for the specific activity you're about to do. Just think about this for a minute though. If you're watching boxing on TV and they show a fighter going through their warm-up in the changing room what do you normally see them doing? Depending on how close they are to the fight you might see them doing activities like shadow-boxing or punching the pads with their trainer. They are warming up the muscles and going through movements they are about to do. If you watch a professional rugby team warming up before a game what would you expect to see there? You'd probably see them practicing line out jumps, going through some running and passing drills with the ball, tackling the bags, the kicker having a few sighters, all movements which they are about to do in their upcoming exercise activity. So how, without trying to shame anyone or any activity in particular, would bending down and touching your toes before going for a run relate to that activity? How would pulling your chin towards your chest to stretch the neck before playing relate to badminton? How would pulling your arm across in front of you to stretch your tricep be an example of recreating a movement relevant to your upcoming bike ride? Like I said, that's not to shame those stretches or activities in particular as I've just picked three activities and thought of three stretches that are wrong, so if you happen to do all of those activities and do all of those stretches then don't feel bad as you're not alone! A warm-up is supposed to prepare our muscles for the upcoming activity. If you were looking to improve how much weight you could lift when squatting would you do a bicep curl as a warm-up? That would seem silly as it bears no resemblance to the activity you're about to do but yet in other activities we happily do warm-up exercises that have nothing to do with what we're about to do.

Looking back at the rugby team warm-up example again the players practice tackling the bags, not each other. The kicker would start with some close simple kicks and then gradually build up to longer, more difficult kicks. They wouldn't walk out on to the pitch in the warm-up, tee it up in the position of the longest, most difficult kick they've ever done in their career and give it their absolute maximum effort to make it with cold, unprepared muscles. This might all seem like it's stating the obvious but if your warm-up for a six-a-side football match consists of running to the pitch from the car park, putting your boots on and then going straight on to the pitch and into the game, are your muscles really ready for football? Before a run if you bend down and touch your toes in the lounge, then pull your heels to your bum to stretch the quads, open the front door and start running as soon as you're past the doorstep, are the muscles really prepared for running? With this in mind we can't go through a suitable warm-up for every exercise or sports activity but you should always aim to recreate movements that you're about to do. This should be done gently initially but, as the warm-up progresses, so can the intensity until you reach the point where you're ready to go.

"I never warm-down. What stretches should I do?"

I think that warm-downs, much like warm-ups, are something that people think they should do but are often either unsure on what to do, don't make time to do them after exercise or maybe have a couple of stretches they quickly do out of courtesy because they think something is better than nothing. Alas, much like stretching when cold, stretching muscles that don't need to be stretched can actually increase your chances of injury rather than reduce them. So, in its simplest form, a warm-down should consist of static stretches that lengthen the muscles that have just been shortened during exercise. That doesn't mean stretch what hurts or copy what everyone else is doing. You need to think about what movements the activity you've just done entailed, what muscles have potentially worked hard and shortened and therefore, which muscles need to be stretched and lengthened. This can often be tricky because, as we've covered countless times throughout the book, short, tight muscles often don't hurt so the temptation is there to stretch out the muscles that do hurt. You might be tempted to stretch your lower back out after a bike ride if it aches but if you've just spent two hours in the saddle leaning forward and stretching your back then it's likely aching because it's already overstretched so stretching it again and more intensely when you finish would make it worse. There are numerous other examples we could talk about here but the common theme would always be to think about how your muscles have worked before jumping to stretch the muscles that ache. If muscles are aching after exercise then, the chances are, they are tired and overstretched so, although stretching them further wouldn't be the answer, using the foam roller could well be of benefit. As I'm sure you can imagine this all leads to a conclusion of a warm-down, much like a warm-up, needing to be specific to the individual activity. For example, a warm-down for after swimming will be different to that for after a run which will differ to that for after tennis.

"Should I use a support/brace/insole?"

There isn't a simple answer to this question as it varies depending upon the issue the individual is presenting with. As a rough guide I generally encourage clients not to use supports unless it's for a reason at the more extreme ends of the scale. At one end of the scale we're looking at new, acute issues where immediate support is needed. Using a support would also usually be accompanied by anti-inflammatories and the use of ice, compression and elevation. A classic example of this would be a twisted ankle where, in the short-term, the support could aid the stability of the joint and allow the individual to start weight-bearing sooner and, as such, increase the speed of recovery. However, it must be said that not all ankle sprains require a support so I have to emphasise that the use of supports is recommended on a case-by-case basis. At the other end of the scale we have situations where a client may have a chronic issue that can't be improved and is just being managed. In some of these cases, psychologically as well as physically, it can be advantageous to use a support for increased confidence when you know an upcoming activity will likely cause stress on an existing issue. Using the ankle as an example, if I have a client with a chronic issue due to previous trauma and/or surgery and we know that there are limitations to the capabilities of the joint, then we might decide on them wearing an ankle support if they are doing a more extreme activity than their normal ones (e.g. a 50K charity walk).

I think in both of those examples that the short-term usage of a support could be beneficial, however, the key part of that statement is 'short-term'. The clue is in the title with the word support itself. They are designed to support you but, with the body there is a fine line between support and reliance. If you wear a support for too long then the body can start to rely on it and, as such, the support becomes counterproductive to your recovery and you end up becoming weaker in the affected area. This in turn actually increases your risk of further injury.

We're designed to be able to support ourselves through being strong and efficient. If an area of the body becomes used to being supported externally then it learns that it doesn't have to support itself and therefore becomes less efficient and weaker. At the time of writing there is currently an influx of upper back braces coming on to the market essentially claiming to cure bad posture and I'm not a fan. Posture improvements are made by gradually releasing off the short, tight muscles and by strengthening up the weak, overstretched muscles – not by wearing a brace. If wearing the brace is the only way your body becomes used to having good posture then you'll be stuck wearing it all day, every day for the rest of your life. On the whole, prolonged wearing of supports/braces/insoles tends to do more harm than good as it discourages your body from supporting itself through strength and efficiency.

However, in the short-term they can have their uses. If your lower back goes into spasm then wearing a back brace for a couple of days might help. If you've twisted your knee and it's ballooned up then, sure, wear a brace for a couple of days if it feels better for wearing it. If your tennis elbow has got so bad that you can't grip things properly then wearing a support for a few days may give you some temporary relief. But these are only temporary measures as they are purely to aid with firefighting the symptom. As soon as you can (according to the severity of the issue) you need to restrengthen/realign to regain the strength, confidence and functionality in the affected area. When it comes to insoles, specifically, I always ask clients to wait until they are as aligned as they can be before committing to anything. Not only could this save them a lot of money but also it once again reduces the risks of becoming reliant on a support. If your body gets used to you having an insole in all your shoes all of the time then what happens when you go barefoot or wear flip-flops? However, if you spend a bit of time working on your strength and alignment before committing to insoles you may well find that your pain is rectified as you have become strong enough to support yourself. I must say here that I have seen a handful examples of short-term insole usage being beneficial and also do have a couple of clients who, due to underlying conditions, do have to wear insoles in all of their footwear and do struggle with walking barefoot. But I have seen many, many more who have either been able to move away from using their insoles all together or have been able to avoid even getting them in the first place by working on their overall strength and alignment.

"Is yoga good for you?"

This is another question that doesn't have a simple yes or no answer as it depends on the individual at the given time. In principle yoga should be good for you as it encourages strength, stability, balance, control and flexibility, all of which generally contribute positively towards an efficient body. The caveat to this though is that yoga is challenging and, as such, I've seen a number of clients over the years where yoga has proved to be a tipping point for them feeling pain or becoming injured. I always tell clients that you need to have a decent base layer of balance, strength and stability before starting out for yoga to be beneficial for you. If not, where a key focus of yoga is working everything equally and in as balanced a way as possible, if you are unknowingly significantly misaligned then sometimes this can accidentally highlight imbalances and make them worse. Say, for example, the hamstrings on one leg are much tighter than the other leg then the pelvis will be slightly rotated and one side of your lower back will be more overstretched than the other side. If you then stretch this further through yoga practice then you could very well, unintentionally, be making the issue worse. The same could be said for an overstretched groin being lengthened further or an inflamed rotator cuff that is taken to a position that it doesn't want to go and accidentally gets further inflamed.

I must stress, by contrast, I have seen a greater number of clients benefit from adding yoga to their list of activities than I have those who have been hindered. Furthermore, you don't have to be perfectly balanced and exceptionally strong for it to be beneficial to you. However, I will often talk to clients about if they're 'good enough' for yoga to help them. Of course, sometimes you just don't know until you try but if you're looking at yoga to be the thing that makes you balanced and strong I would always advise seeing or chatting to someone professional beforehand just to make sure that it will definitely benefit you. One final point with yoga is that, although we can all potentially make improvements with our flexibility by practising it, I strongly believe that balance and efficiency are more important than flexibility. You might be someone who can try until they turn blue in the face to touch your toes but it's just not going to happen and yet you can still be equal. Conversely, you might be able to touch your toes comfortably but have one hamstring much tighter than the other and, as such, be at a higher risk of injury due to your imbalance. The point here is that we all have different capabilities so as long as you're in tune with your body and make improvements by your standards that's what counts.

"Is pilates good for you?"

Again, in principle pilates is good for you but, much like with yoga, it does depend massively on where an individual is starting from in terms of functionality and balance. The principles of strength, stability and balance are fundamental to pilates but, as per the case with yoga, if you are significantly imbalanced in the first place then strengthening and challenging everything equally may not be what your body needs. If you are imbalanced then strengthening one side more than the other would be required to balance you up so, consequently, working both sides equally won't achieve this. Also, if an exercise in pilates is too difficult for you the chances are that, as is usually the case with the body, other muscles will take over and you may accidentally find yourself doing the movement correctly but by using the wrong muscles. The most frequent example of this is occurs when the glutes aren't quite strong enough and then the hamstrings take over. Although it may well look like you're doing the exercise correctly, if this were the case then you could inadvertently be shortening the hamstrings, while at the same time inhibiting glute functionality which in turn adds more stress to your hips and lower back.

In comparison to yoga injuries, I've only seen a handful of clients where pilates has made them worse but I do get asked about it a lot so I thought it was worth a mention. However, by comparing pilates to yoga in this way I'm not suggesting that pilates is better for you than yoga. In my clinical experience I have seen less people have issues due to the stress of pilates compared to yoga but I firmly believe that, as long as the individual is equal and strong enough in the first place, both can be beneficial towards your physical and mental wellbeing.

CHAPTER 10

A Few Final Thoughts

There isn't really a conclusion to this book because there's nothing conclusive about the body. We're in a constant state of change and adaptation so there can't be one rule that applies to all situations. However, I feel that there are a few themes and ideas that can act as a guide so hopefully they've been made clear throughout the book and you'll find these useful for the present and the future.

There's no harm drilling home a few of these points one last time so here's a reminder of the principles we've talked about right from the beginning:

- Pain is just the symptom.
- If it hurts don't stretch it.
- If something is overstretched then something else is too short.
- Stretching feels nice but make sure you're stretching the muscle that needs it.

Using these principles as a basis for trying to understand your discomfort will hopefully make a significant difference to how you view and react to pain in your life. When you really think about it you are the only one who is responsible for looking after your body, so the better you get to know and understand it the better chance you have of getting to enjoy its wonderous capabilities.

The idea isn't to ignore pain but to understand it, be curious about it and aim to work out what's actually going on.

Our bodies are incredible but they're not great at telling us the whole story. When something hurts and we experience pain as a symptom we are, more often than not, just being told the end of the story or the end of the dot-to-dot. As such, we can get drawn into focusing on the symptom and trying to change it when, in reality, a change elsewhere in the network is what is required to resolve the issue. Any time you feel pain I want you to think, "Why does that hurt?" Just taking a moment to question why the pain may have occurred is the game changer. Rather than automatically stretching or rubbing what hurts, you have to manually override the system by hitting the pause button and giving yourself a moment to try and figure out the chain of events that could have caused the issue.

Don't put pressure on yourself to figure everything out on your own

You can't be expected to self-diagnose every issue that you have. I've been doing this for over a decade and I'm still learning and developing every day because you can't possibly know everything in this field. However, when you do experience discomfort, not doing the wrong thing is more of a positive step than inadvertently making things worse. Even if you don't know what the right thing to do is at least not making things worse is beneficial. I got into this field because I knew that stretching certain things was making me feel worse but I didn't know what I should stretch instead.

Hopefully, this book has given you some examples and ideas to help you with this but, as I've said throughout, if in doubt always seek professional support.

Don't put pressure on yourself to instantly break habits

If you do lean on one leg more than the other when you stand then you can't expect to change this overnight. If you cross your legs when you sit it's not realistic to expect yourself to suddenly stop doing it now you're aware of it because it could be a habit that's been going on for years.

There's only one you and your body

No one else in this world has your injury history, sofa, car, job, hobbies, interests, genes etc. So that's why there can't be a concrete set of rules for how to use your body. At various stages of life your body will enjoy different things. At various stages of the day your body will enjoy different things. You have to get to know your body and it doesn't really matter what anyone else can do because they're not you. I hope that you've got some new ideas from this book that inspire you to understand your body even more.

This isn't about aiming for a perfect posture because there's no such thing. It's about making your body function the best that it can so that you can get the most out of it and live your life enjoying exploring its wonderous capabilities.

Lightning Source UK Ltd.
Milton Keynes UK
UKHW010641130522
402944UK00002B/291